Planning for a Healthy Baby

Foresight

The Association for the Promotion of Preconceptual Care

Planning for a Healthy Baby

Belinda Barnes
and
Suzanne Gail Bradley

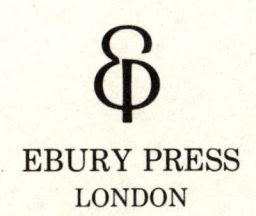

EBURY PRESS
LONDON

First published by Ebury Press
an imprint of Century Hutchinson Ltd
20 Vauxhall Bridge Road
London SW1V 2SA

Copyright © 1990 Belinda Barnes and Suzanne Gail Bradley

All rights reserved. No part of the publication may be reproduced, stored in a retrieval system, or transmitted in any form or by any means, electronic, mechanical, photocopying, recording or otherwise, without the prior permission of the copyright owners.

British Library Cataloguing in Publication Data
Barnes, Belinda
  Foresight: planning for a healthy baby.
  1. Women. Pregnancy. Health aspects
  I. Title II. Bradley, Suzanne Gail
  618.2'4

ISBN 0-85223-850-9

Typeset by Textype Typesetters, Cambridge
Printed and bound by Mackays of Chatham PLC

DEDICATION

This book is dedicated to the memories of the late
Lilian Schofield, a pioneer in the wholefood
movement, the late Dr Carl Pfeiffer, a leading
expert on nutritional biochemistry, and to
Dr Elizabeth Lodge-Rees, whose work has been so
influential in the development of Foresight.

FORESIGHT

Foresight is a registered charity and was formed in 1978 as the Association for the Promotion of Pre-Conceptual Care. It also promotes research into the harmful effects of factors in the environment upon Fetal Development.

If you need further advice or the address of your nearest Foresight clinician please write, enclosing an s.a.e., to Foresight, The Old Vicarage, Witley, Godalming, Surrey GU8 5PN.

WARNING

This book gives non-specific, general advice. You should consult your own doctor or a Foresight clinician for individual assessment and treatment.

ACKNOWLEDGEMENTS

This book could not have been written without the help of our friends, colleagues and advisers. We are especially indebted to Sir Richard Body, Professor Derek Bryce-Smith, Marion Cashman, Dr Stephen Davies, Dr Damien Downing, Jennifer Edwards, Dr Ellen Grant, Dr Patrick Kingsley, Mary Langman, Jennifer Masefield, Eve Mervin-Smith, Dr Michael Nightingale, Colleen Norman, Dr Grahame Sutton, Dr Neil Ward and Margaret and Arthur Wynn. Any errors are ours.

Contents

INTRODUCTION

The Basic FORESIGHT Plan

PART ONE: FORESIGHT
- page 12   Chapter 1   The Beginnings of Foresight
- page 20   Chapter 2   Foresight Case Histories

PART TWO: THE NEED FOR INTERVENTION
- page 34   Chapter 3   Preconception Care

PART THREE: POSITIVE STEPS FOR HEALTHY OFFSPRING
- page 46   Chapter 4   The Preconception Medical Check – the Foresight Way
- page 54   Chapter 5   The Vital Role of Nutrition in Pregnancy
- page 76   Chapter 6   Planning Your Family the Natural Way

PART FOUR: NEGATIVE INFLUENCES ON PRECONCEPTION AND PRENATAL HEALTH
- page 82   Chapter 7   Problems in the Twentieth Century: Toxic Metals
- page 93   Chapter 8   Problems in the Twentieth Century: Drugs
- page 103   Chapter 9   Problems in the Twentieth Century: Harmful Contraception Methods
- page 111   Chapter 10   Physical and Chemical Hazards in the Workplace and Home
- page 122   Chapter 11   Food Production
- page 135   Chapter 12   Food-related Illness
- page 145   Chapter 13   Diseases
- page 154   Chapter 14   Tests During Pregnancy
- page 160   Chapter 15   Postscript

- page 163   Glossary
- page 165   Appendix One   List of Useful Addresses
- page 168   Appendix Two   Recommended Reading List
- page 169   Appendix Three   Food Allergy Questionnaire
- page 174   References
- page 186   Index

Introduction
by Belinda Barnes

There is no more daunting moment than when, having rolled a pristine sheet of paper into the typewriter, the first sentence of a new book remains elusive...Luckily at this stage the telephone rings:

'I've had the baby! Four days ago – and she's lovely, absolutely perfect! She was due today so she was just a little bit early...8 lb 8 oz. I wish you could see her...quite a lot of fair hair and her eyes are dark like the others were, they'll get paler and be blue, I expect. She's such a pretty baby and her brother and sister think she's wonderful, which is lucky. It only took two hours from start to finish. I was amazed – we only just made it to the hospital! The placenta was very healthy, they said a healthy placenta makes a healthy baby...it makes sense...and really she is. All the midwives have been admiring her – I can't thank you enough.'

'Well, I'm thrilled for you, but don't thank me; you did it all.'

'No, but we think it was due to Foresight...all the advice and supplements and that, we think that's why she's so gorgeous. Louisa Jane, we're calling her...I'll be in touch next year. It makes you want another when they're so lovely, doesn't it? My husband will go mad if he hears me!'

Bless you, Louisa Jane. What could be a more auspicious introduction to a book on preconceptual care?

Why, when and where did preconceptual care and the setting up of Foresight first start? The birth of an idea is not like the birth of a baby, full of energy and triumph, but unfolds gradually from past experience, the gathering of relevant knowledge and, in this case, from a feeling of certainty that babies were not meant to be born dead, malformed, mentally afflicted, frail, sickly or disadvantaged in any way. The founders of Foresight were all mothers who had known the magical happiness of giving birth, and that enriching experience plus basic commonsense and the enlightening research of others was the spur that drove us onwards.

This book is the sum of nearly ten years of knowledge from working with parents and babies towards a safer and happier future and includes material on the background research upon which our ideas are based.

It is intended as a book for mothers and fathers, for doctors, midwives and health visitors who are promoting positive health, and for research scientists. References are given for those who want to study the subject of preconceptual care in depth.

But above all, this book is written for the ordinary couple who want a healthy family, to give them some of the hard facts they need to circumnavigate the complicated minefield of environmental pollution, chemical hazards, inadequate foods, apathy and misinformation that exists. Foresight believes the fullest possible information on health matters gives people the chance to help their families and in no area is it so imperative that there is access to detailed information as in the area of reproductive health. As one Cambridge researcher points out:

> Hormonal and vitamin imbalances which can cause malaise or even pass unnoticed in postnatal life may have a disastrous effect on the developing fetus...interference with growth or metabolism of developing cells at an early stage is reflected ultimately in alterations at the stage of differentiation with resulting malformations or impaired function of developing organs and tissues...As a rule, the demands of the mother for vitamins take priority over fetal demands, so that in many cases there may be no sign of maternal deficiency in essential food factors, while at the same time the fetus may be suffering marked deficiency. This means that a marginal maternal deficiency, which is very difficult to detect, may have grave consequences for the fetus.[1]

Research and our own experience, however, lead us to believe that most of the damage and ill-health that afflicts the unborn can be pre-empted if certain measures are taken in time. We also know from the letters Foresight receives that parents who have had problems are losing patience with remarks such as: 'Better luck next time', 'We'll keep our fingers crossed for you', 'There was nothing you could have done', 'Nobody knows why these things happen' and other verbal tranquillisers.

The first part of the book examines the history and work of Foresight and includes many case histories from parents who have followed the Foresight programme. In the second part we explain the reasons why pre-pregnancy planning is essential. In the third part we explore the positive steps you can take to optimise the baby's chances of normal healthy development. Part four describes the negative influences on this healthy development and how best their effects may be avoided or minimised.

BELINDA BARNES
1989

The Basic FORESIGHT Plan

The basic plan is that six months prior to the intended conception both partners should:

- Eat a good wholefood diet, free from dangerous additives, and organically produced wherever possible. Additives can be checked out with the little pocketbook, *Find Out*, available from Foresight (£1.35 inc p&p). *The Foresight Wholefood Cookbook* has over 400 recipes and advice on nutrition (£6.25 inc p&p). For names of organic suppliers in your locality, join Foresight and your Branch Secretary can let you know.
- Use natural family planning (fertility awareness) with abstention or barrier methods during the fertile period. The fertile period is the five days preceding ovulation and the day you ovulate. The address of your nearest natural family planning teacher can be supplied by your Foresight Branch Secretary.
- Have mineral analyses done, and follow the programme of supplementation and cleansing as indicated. Retest as advised, and do not conceive until the toxic metals have been cleansed, and the levels of essential minerals optimised.
- Use a Waymaster Crystal water filter.
- Check for rubella status, toxoplasmosis, allergies, malabsorption and candida albicans, and have any immunisation, treatment or adapt the diet as advised. Clearing up allergies by dietary maniplulation may eliminate the need for some drugs.
- Have a colposcopy examination to check for genito-urinary infection, and seek treatment necessary. If there is infection present, see your partner is also treated. After treatment, retest.
- Eliminate alcohol, smoking and all but absolutely necessary medical drugs. Check with your GP that any drugs you are taking are not contraindicated in pregnancy.
- Avoid the use of organophosphate pesticides in the home, or materials treated with pesticides.
- Read this book, and use the information we have gathered together for you to have a successful and very happy pregnancy!

PART ONE

Foresight

CHAPTER 1

The Beginnings of Foresight

HOW WE CAME INTO BEING — WHY WE CAME INTO BEING — AND HOW WE HOPE WE CAN HELP YOU.

In the late 1960s I (Belinda Barnes) was seeking help for the treatment of coeliac condition, hyperactivity and dyslexia in my own family which led to my reading the *Journal of Orthomolecular Psychiatry*. An article in that journal described the problems of the allergic, dyslexic child so perceptively, and the whole made so much sense that I decided to contact the author, Dr Lodge-Rees, and invite her to England to speak and to bring me what information she could.

Dr Elizabeth Lodge-Rees flew into Heathrow one memorable dawn. 'I've got arms the length of an orang-utan, honey, from carting all those darned books in my hand-luggage. You have to look nonchalant or they weigh things and charge you extra baggage – I've nearly dislocated both shoulders!'

The hand-luggage contained education for life! Among those 'darned books' were Dr Weston Price's epic *Nutrition and Physical Degeneration*, the works of that brilliant and witty nutritionist Dr Roger Williams, Wilfred Shute on Vitamin E, Linus Pauling on Vitamin C and Carl Pfeiffer on trace minerals. Despite having Beth as a house guest I read until 4.30 am that night. I thought then, and later I still think, that Dr Weston Price's book should be read by everyone concerned with human health, and particularly with human reproduction. His empirical findings will stand for all time. Analytical methods available to him in the 30s were not as sophisticated as those available today, and there are environmental hazards around now, which were not around in his time. But the basic discoveries of the roots of human health in wholefood and in the soil on which the food was grown will remain, and each generation will be able to scrutinise these and come up with their own interpretations, as knowledge advances.

Interest in the potential of this work, and that of Lodge-Rees, McCarrison, Pfeiffer, Williams, Jennings and others, led me to involvement with a wide variety of voluntary organisations. They were concerned with allergic illness, deficiency diseases and environmental problems of all kinds. These organisations were scouring the world for information, and trying to get together the funds to finance research.

In the mid-1970s, many in the medical profession regarded allergic illness and deficiency syndromes as a thoroughly 'suspect area' and preferred to think most of the symptoms were of 'mental origin'. The influence of Freud still existed, although his theories had been much adapted and manipulated down the years. Most doctors still relied heavily on their formal training and the examination system discouraged lateral thought. There was a heavy emphasis on increasing knowledge via the convention of the double-blind trial. This is thought to be necessary as it is sometimes believed that many spontaneous remissions take place due solely to the charisma of the doctor involved.

Be that as it may, the obvious disadvantage of this approach is that it inhibits the introduction of almost any new ideas, save those concerned with the use of drugs (or, more rarely, with vitamins and minerals), as only pills or capsules easily lend themselves to the provision of identical placebos. These trials are mainly funded by the drug companies and information is disseminated at conferences, and/or through medical journals, the more popular of which are largely funded by advertisements provided by the drug companies.

Greater numbers of doctors and research scientists are now becoming increasingly concerned by the limitations of this approach. Deficiencies, especially of zinc, are receiving more attention, and allergies, sensitivities or idiosyncratic reactions to foods and other substances are being considered more thoughtfully. These deficiencies can usually be tracked backwards to a poor diet of inadequate 'junk' food, to slimming regimes, to over-use of agrochemicals, to the manipulation of biochemistry by artificial hormones, to environmental poisons, and to chronic infection of the genito-urinary tract. Gradually ecological medicine looks more credible.

We are all more aware of some tragic medical mishaps that have taken place despite trials – thalidomide, opren, the benzodiazepines. We have also become much more aware of trials that were NOT done in the past regarding the dangers of tobacco, lead, mercury, additives, pesticides and alcohol, for example.

In the 70s therefore, the founders of Foresight were still discussing all of these issues, tracing the source of problems and piecing together the jigsaw with the information from books, research papers and from the collective experience of many voluntary organisations. Over time the links between environmental fecklessness and the daily sagas of family trials and tragedies emerged more clearly. This revealed an urgent need for prevention and at the end of the 70s, there seemed to be a lot that could be achieved if only information and help could be got to people in time. The writers, Arthur and Margaret Wynn, well-known authorities on fetal health and development, had collected together a lot of data from post-war Europe, which demonstrated that the crucial period for successful reproduction is the four months prior to conception. The sperm and the ovum are vulnerable as they grow and develop. It seemed that to be effective we had to think about the time *before* conception.

The five of us who had been involved from the beginning of Foresight were a community health council secretary, a midwife, a nutritionist, a supporter of the Cheshire Homes Charity and an ex-nursery nurse. We talked over the feasibility of preconceptual care. We knew doctors and research workers who were involved with the voluntary organisations. In those days they were quite a select band, although now they are quite an army. We talked our ideas over with them, and it was from among them we found the first doctors with the knowledge and the commitment to pioneer preconceptual care. In October 1978, with their help, we started Foresight.

The doctors were, in the main, interested in nutritional medicine and in environmental and food allergies. Some had made a study of homeopathy, and some were women doctors with a particular interest in mothers and small children.

Beth Lodge-Rees came over several times to teach the interpretation of hair analysis. In the first few years we held meetings which included her, Professor Carl Pfeiffer and Dr Oberleas. Their work convinced the Foresight team of the vital role of trace elements. At first it was necessary to send hair samples to an American laboratory, but some years later, analysis became available in this country. Sweat and blood analyses are also used and research continues.

The Work of Foresight

Because not all of the Foresight protocol is available on the NHS, Foresight clinicians have to do the work privately. For this reason we took a lot of flak at the beginning from people telling us preconceptual care would become a 'fad' for rich women who had nothing better to do. Foresight experience down the years has been entirely different from this with people coming to us from a wide variety of backgrounds.

Infertility

One of the largest groups is of couples coming with problems associated with fertility. Women come with unexplained infertility, or with known problems, including blocked Fallopian tubes, amenorrhoea, anovulation, polycystic ovaries and endometriosis.

When they are given the full Foresight check-up (see Chapter 4) the clinician often finds they suffer from nutritional deficiencies, high toxic metals, or over-high copper, allergies, malabsorption, candida albicans, and often an unsuspected genito-urinary infection. Diet may have been inadequate. Smoking and alcohol may have to be discontinued.

High copper and low zinc, often with low magnesium and/or manganese, are the commonest findings, and this is usually after use of the pill or the copper coil. Low zinc lays people open to infections of all types, and it is common for chlamydia and mycoplasmas to be involved. Work at Surrey University has found the high copper/low zinc syndrome to alter the secretions in the Fallopian tubes, and this may render them more vulnerable to adhesions infection.

When zinc levels are fully restored and general health is much improved, ovulation and menstruation will often restart naturally. Sometimes people are impatient, however, and opt for Clomid, and where this happens after a partial Foresight programme, they will often find the smallest possible dose will restore ovulation. It has not been unknown for people with supposedly blocked tubes to become pregnant while waiting for surgery or IVF (In-Vitro Fertilisation). This is probably where the blocking was catarrhal from allergy or infection or the wall of the tube was oedematose, possibly due to allergy. Tubes said to be atrophied or twisted can sometimes revive with improved health. However, where there are severe adhesions, surgery may be necessary. If so, improved general health and adequate Vitamins C and E and zinc will make clean healing more likely with less scar tissue.

Sperm problems
We hear from quite a lot of men (or from their wives) who suffer from poor sperm health, manifesting as a low count, poor motility or malformations. Sometimes they have been told that adoption or AID is the only answer, but at Foresight we have found that measures taken to optimise the health of the man will usually improve the health of the sperm. As always, we suggest the full Foresight programme. Zinc, manganese, Vitamins E and B12 have been reported as especially important to a good count. Adequate thyroid function has also been found vital. Potassium has been reported to increase motility. We pay particular attention to these factors. The dropping of alcohol and smoking have been found to improve counts dramatically. Contamination with lead is known to produce malformed sperm. We suggest avoiding hot baths and tight clothing. It is essential to check for genito-urinary infections. Organophosphate pesticides should be avoided.

We have been told that testicular cancer, controlled by radiotherapy, leaves permanent sterility, but in other situations we remain hopeful as we have frequently found our regime has proved successful.

We are sometimes asked about antibody problems after a reversed vasectomy. Two fathers have successfully had a child and one has had two. However, we do advise very strongly against vasectomy in young men, as they seem so often to change their mind, and reversal can be difficult.

We have had several couples where the woman has been said to have 'hostile mucus' or to be making antibodies to her husband's sperm. We have found either an infection in the husband, or a very high level of toxic metal. We surmise (no more!) that if the sperm are not in good condition, the woman's body may make efforts to destroy them. It would therefore always seem worthwhile, before trying other things, to have a full Foresight check-up and programme.

Miscarriage
Another large group who come to us are the couples who have suffered one or many miscarriage(s). One mother came to us having had seven, then we achieved Sally... After the full Foresight programme it is very rare indeed for there to be another miscarriage. In many cases we find a problem in the father and it may be that many more miscarriages are due to poor sperm health than is usually acknowledged.

Neo-natal death
Another sad group who come to us are those who have lost a baby at birth or soon after birth. Some of these deaths may be due to a difficult labour or birth accident. Many of the mothers have suffered pre-eclamptic toxaemia, and the baby has been brought on too early to sustain life. Some of the babies have been born with a malformation incompatible with life.

The Foresight programme seems to have been helpful with mothers who have had threatened pre-eclamptic toxaemia, or have just had high blood pressure with previous pregnancies. That may be because we correct low zinc levels, or clear the toxic metals, particularly cadmium. There may have been allergies, or perhaps it is because giving big doses of Vitamin C helped to lessen the pesticide contamination. Pesticides interfere with choline metabolism and choline is vital to liver function. For whatever reason, the Foresight pregnancy usually goes better, although sometimes the baby has to be born a week or two early.

Malformations
Some couples contact us because there has been a cluster of malformations in the geographical location where they live. This is very worrying. We try to help them trace drinking water problems, factory effluent, pesticide use, heavy motorway pollution or other possible problems. Hair analysis can be helpful, as it can show up metal pollution. We try to help them work out a solution.

Many couples come to us with a little disabled child, who has managed to overcome his/her problem and live. I am always inspired by their courage and cheerfulness. 'We wouldn't change him for the world,' they say, 'but next time, we would love to have the baby without the problem.' Many malformations seem to be due to deficiencies, and others may be due to toxic metals or infection. We advise the full Foresight programme for both partners, and we have never had another malformation, although two mothers have come to us previously having had two children with problems, and one mother with coeliac condition had had three. One of the most common anomalies in the 1980s is undescended testicles. This may follow pill use in the mother and may be at least partly due to zinc deficiency. This is one more reason why it is important to drop artificial hormones well in advance of the pregnancy and make sure your zinc levels are good.

Older mothers

A lot of mothers come to us because they believe they are 'old' to be planning a pregnancy, and some are over 40 years of age. With some, it is an addition to the family, with others this will be the first pregnancy. In many cases they are being discouraged by relatives and friends from embarking on a pregnancy. We give them information and try not to influence the decision, but each time it gets harder to be objective, when we see how splendid the babies are, and how good the older mums are at coping!

We take particular care with selenium levels in our older parents, as Down's syndrome has been linked to low levels of selenium in research done in the USA.

It has to be said, however, that where there are fertility problems with older parents, when the mother is in her forties it can be harder to resolve, so we do suggest coming to us a little earlier if circumstances permit.

General health

Quite a lot of prospective parents come to us with health problems of their own. Eczema, asthma, migraine, epilepsy and diabetes are common. Some are suffering from insomnia or depression that is being treated by drugs upon which they may have become dependent. Some have been on the pill and have side-effects which they may or may not recognise as such. Some have discharge, vaginal pain or irritation, back pain or pain on urinating. Some may have been told the discharge is functional and nothing to worry about, although it may mean genito-urinary infection. They may suffer, or have suffered, from minor problems such as short-sight, orthodontal problems, squints, or from quite major handicaps like club feet, cleft palate or similar. Some are worried by their dependency on tobacco, alcohol, or a more dangerous drug. Others had problems with a previous pregnancy such as hyperemesis (excessive sickness and vomiting), pre-eclamptic toxaemia or high blood pressure, a long slow labour, lactation failure or postnatal depression.

In some instances it is the relatives who get in touch with us as they are worried. If this is mother-in-law agonising about a daughter-in-law's smoking or poor eating habits, this may need very careful handling! Often it is a heartbroken mother or sister concerned about miscarriage, or infertility. We tell them about our work in great detail to give them renewed hope, and send them all the information we have.

Quite a lot of mothers contact us well into their pregnancy, having only just heard of us, or because there is a problem, such as hyperemesis, high blood pressure, fatigue or sleeplessness. We give what help we can but, as we know the troubles may stem from some months prior to conception, we do like to see people sooner if possible.

Quite a number of Foresight mothers who have had a lot of sickness with previous pregnancies tell us they got on much better with the Foresight pregnancy. One mother who had been hospitalised with hyperemesis in two previous pregnancies wrote with triumph that she had only been sick six times during ours! Many seem to make it through without succumbing at all. With this, high blood pressure and with excessive fatigue, I think it is probably the combination of cleansing the toxins and supplementing the vitamins and zinc, in particular, which seems to help. For fatigue, kelp for iodine and Vitamin C helps.

For varicose veins we suggest selenium, Vitamins E and C.

Premature labour seems to be very tied in with high copper, as Vallee's work would suggest. When there has been a previous small baby/premature birth we try to get the zinc well up and the copper well within the normal range.

Work with cows and sheep in Australia indicates that a strong vigorous labour is encouraged by plenty of zinc, so we see the zinc level is well up, and there is plenty of Vitamin E which encourages elasticity of the tissues.

Generally the Foresight post-partum experience is good. Almost no mothers have suffered from post-partum depression. We encourage them to maintain a good level of zinc, manganese, magnesium, B-Complex vitamins and essential fatty acids. Deficiency of any of these is known to make people prone to depression unless some supplementation is taken. Where there is enough zinc and Vitamins C, E and A, the healing of any abrasions of the vagina or of an episiotomy should be cleaner and less painful and sore breasts and cracked nipples should not occur. We also give calcium and Vitamin D as these are said to encourage sleep and perhaps this is one of the reasons we keep hearing how good and calm the Foresight babies are. Zinc and manganese encourage maternal bonding, and repletion in all essential nutrients makes for good quality breast milk. We believe the quality is as important as the quantity, and this seems to have been borne out as almost every Foresight mother has breastfed – many for over a year.

Where the baby is contented, bonding is much closer, not only with the mother, but with the father and siblings as well. A 'good' baby is a great joy and a great relief all round!

Where breastfeeding is steady, weaning can be a slow gentle process, going at the baby's own pace, and this helps to combat allergy – although there are, as we know, a lot of other factors involved.

What happens when you contact Foresight?

We send a letter of welcome, the name of the nearest Foresight clinician to where you live and our explanatory leaflet. We are delighted if you join the organisation, as this helps us to run our research projects, keeps us going, and helps you to keep in touch with what is going on regarding Foresight. You will then be put in touch with your Branch Secretary and you will be invited to attend talks as and when they occur. She will be able to supply the names of local organic food suppliers, or mail order firms, and your nearest

Natural Family Planning teacher. She may also know where you can obtain lead-free petrol locally and which cars run on it, and how/whether your car can be adapted. She can advise you on books on the background research, and/or let you know if there are talks on preconceptual care and allied subjects given by the group. We send three newsletters a year to all members to disseminate news and results from our research projects.

Please send an SAE when you write to us. Our address is FORESIGHT, The Old Vicarage, Church Lane, Witley, Godalming, Surrey GU8 5PN.

The leaflet has a list of Foresight books and booklets, including *The Foresight Wholefood Cookbook*. This gives a lot of useful information on diet and choosing foods, and ways of cooking to preserve the vitamin and mineral content, as well as over 400 recipes. There is also *Find Out*, our pocket guide for checking out which are the harmful additives.

If your own GP has an interest in preparing couples for pregnancy, and is knowledgeable in the areas covered in Chapter 4, he/she may be willing to give a check-up as outlined.

Your Foresight clinician, who sees patients privately, will have made a particular study of allergies, malabsorption, candida and mineral metabolism, and can advise you on infections, diet and lifestyles, and arrange any necessary medical tests.

If any doctor is reading this book who believes in preventative care and creating a healthier population in a healthier environment, please contact us and see whether you would like to join us. You are very welcome. We need more help.

CHAPTER 2

Foresight Case Histories

HOW SOME OF YOU USED THE EXTRA HELP AND INFORMATION TO TRIUMPH OVER ADVERSITY.

Writing about Foresight case histories, it is hard to know where to start. I will focus on the mothers who come to us with a problem, or after a tragedy, and whose baby has arrived so I know the outcome of the Foresight pregnancy. There is not room for a lot of detail, and some of the particulars are disguised so not to breach our confidentiality.

Nevertheless, there is plenty to send us all on our way rejoicing.

Infertility

An important group we hear from are those suffering from infertility. Sometimes they are trying for their first baby, sometimes they have one child, but a brother or sister is not forthcoming so they contact us.

A case of lead in the water?
Mr and Mrs J.F. wrote to us from a Scottish city, known to us for the lead in the water. They had been trying for a baby for over four years. Hair analysis revealed a towering lead level in both partners, and Mrs J.F. also had a very high copper level, and low zinc, manganese and other essential minerals. She was a lactovegetarian (which can mean less zinc in the diet) and many years before had been using the contraceptive pill. The toxic metals were so high that programmes of cleansing and supplementing went on for over a year, but their patience was finally rewarded. Their little boy was born, weighing 6 lb 14 oz, in 1985. Recently, they have planned another child and have sent hair for analysis again. This was wise, as with Mr J.F. the lead has crept back quite significantly. At work he drinks tea made with unfiltered water, and this spells trouble in this area.

Probable zinc deficiency?
One of our jollier ladies who was waiting for a baby to put in an appearance had a problem with her weight – it kept falling – and she was not menstruating or ovulating. Her Foresight clinician

guessed a zinc deficiency would account for all three problems. Her hair and sweat tests confirmed this and showed quite a lot of other deficient minerals as well. Her clinician helped her to identify the foods to which she was allergic, which included the gluten grains. Many of us might envy her this particular weight problem, but it was a great trial to her, as she knew she had to work very hard to build herself up for the pregnancy. She was aiming for 8½ stone, but fate intervened and the pregnancy started when she was just over 8 stone. She stuck with the Foresight programme and was given help from a homeopathic doctor for the duration of the pregnancy. Her daughter was born weighing 7 lb 6 oz and the doctors were amazed she was such a big baby.

A happy beginning

On another occasion we had a happy beginning. One couple were waiting for artificial insemination by the husband (AIH) to help to solve their fertility problem because the sperm were not sufficiently mobile to reach the egg. We advised them to postpone this until their very common problem of a high level of copper and a low level of zinc had been solved. They had completed their Foresight programme and were waiting for their appointment for AIH when the wife happily realised she was pregnant! In due course their little son of 7 lb 5½ oz arrived. They wrote: 'We took all the sound advice and it was definitely worth it!'

A fraction of an ovary

Mrs D.S. first got in touch when her medical advisers had told her there was no hope of a pregnancy. After surgery, she was left with only a fraction of one ovary. This, they said, had been left so she need not go through the menopause at such a young age. She was also told her tubes had atrophied and twisted and would not function. Her Foresight clinician agreed there was nothing against following a Foresight programme and getting 100 per cent fit, but warned she must not be disappointed if there was no pregnancy. When her baby daughter (7 lb 14 oz) arrived her gynaecologist told her this was a chance in a million, she must not hope it would ever be repeated; this was a miracle baby. But he reckoned without Mrs D.S. and two years later she was back with a second miracle baby, a little sister weighing 7 lb 3 oz.

Another little drink?

Mrs L.R.O. contacted us because she was 35 and wanted to start a family. Her chart showed quite high lead and mercury and she made efforts to trace the source and to get the levels down. Then her husband's job took them abroad for some years and we heard no more. Returning to England, she was disappointed that no pregnancy had happened in the interim. Tests by the NHS on her husband's fertility were disappointing and adoption or AID was suggested. They were both very upset, and she tried to persuade him to have hair, blood and sweat analysis with a Foresight clinician, but he was unwilling to take things further. He did, however, agree to drop his usual two drinks a day, and even this small concession meant that in three months the picture was much improved. Mrs O., meanwhile, continued to keep herself in ace condition (as women will!) and within just a few months there was a pregnancy. Their little boy was 7 lb 6 oz. 'He sucks like a trooper and is very handsome,' we were told.

Allergies and mineral imbalance
Another lady suffering from hay fever and fibroids rang us. She had the low zinc and high copper that often spells out both a tendency to allergies (zinc helps the immune system) and to gynaecological complications. She was advised to leave off eating 'the big grasses' (wheat, rye, oats and barley), as this often helps hay fever, and to take supplements to rebalance her minerals. As she was aged 40, she did not want to postpone the conception, but apart from this, she did everything her clinician suggested. Almost immediately she started her pregnancy, which progressed to 35½ weeks. (High copper and fibroids often means an early birth.) Her son was 4 lb 14 oz, but he was, as his mother said, 'a born fighter and a ferocious sucker', and all went well.

DIY Foresight programme
Mrs B.M. wrote from rural Ireland. She was sad about having infertility problems and wondered if we could help. Hair analysis showed she had no toxic metals, but some essential minerals were low. We had no clinician in her part of Ireland, but she improved her diet and took supplements and in the following year, she had a little girl of 8 lb 14 oz. 'She is such a happy baby and so full of self esteem!' we were told.

A lady from the far north of England wrote saying she suffered from anovulation, but could not afford to see a Foresight clinician. Dietary reform, with Vitamin C to combat toxins from the drinking water, and Foresight vitamins and minerals and zinc may have done the trick, as a few months later a pregnancy started, and along came a little boy of 7 lb 4 oz.

A high mercury level
Mrs J.G.F. from the north-west contacted us after 21 months of infertility and problems with a polyp. She was a dental nurse and her hair analysis revealed rather high levels of mercury. She had previously had to have a termination for malformation. Since contacting Foresight and clearing the mercury, she has had two little girls of 5 lb 9 oz and 6 lb 10 oz.

Complicated problems
A rather complicated history was Mrs C.D. who came to us after trying for a baby for a number of years. She had problems with

intestinal candida, a sensitivity to the gluten grains and a nasty virus. She felt very ill and depressed. Under one of our clinicians, her problems were all sorted out and the conception took place almost straight away. Her little girl was born 7 lb 10½ oz and was described to us as 'beautiful and perfect'. One midwife told her mother, 'This is what all babies should be like, but one so seldom sees it nowadays.' At her postnatal, her GP, who had been so sceptical, said to her, 'Well, that Foresight business was well worth it, wasn't it?'

Mrs G.I., aged 37 years, from the West Country, wrote after eight years of infertility. She suffered from irritable bowel syndrome and intermittent diarrhoea. Her Foresight clinician sorted out her food allergies and corrected her many mineral deficiencies, and she had 'a beautiful healthy little girl who sleeps well', weighing 7 lb 10½ oz.

Two other ladies have come to us who have had irritable bowel syndrome and suffered from infertility. Both conceived successfully once their allergies and candidiasis had been sorted out, and this has meant three more Foresight babies – two boys and a girl.

Hostile mucus
A couple whose home had been in Devon, but who had now come to live in the Home Counties, had a difficult problem with the wife's hostile mucus destroying the husband's sperm. Years before, she had had one very early miscarriage, and since then they had not been able to conceive. We saw a hair chart, and the high lead typical of the West Country (lead waterpipes) was evident. This is not often seen in the Home Counties, where the water is much harder and so does not leach metal from the pipes. Lead is known to cause malformation of sperm. We had a hunch that the mucus might be destroying the damaged sperm, so we cleansed the lead from both of them, and since then two robust little boys (7 lb 11 oz and 7 lb 12 oz) have put in an appearance, with only 16 months between them.

Mrs H.R. came to us with the same problem: her mucus was destroying her husband's sperm. Hair analysis showed a very high level of lead and aluminium in both partners – so we were hopeful. Once cleared, we were soon told that she was pregnant and along came a very big girl, 9 lb 3 oz!

Late pregnancy
It is not at all uncommon for a couple to come to us when the woman has been following an absorbing career for a long time, and then in her late thirties the very well-planned pregnancy does not materialise.

Mrs L.Y. was 39 years when she contacted us. She was suffering from ulcerative colitis, intestinal candida, constant fatigue and fainting. All this, when she had planned to start her family! The happy combined operations of the Foresight clinician who worked out her allergies, the necessary supplements, and the Vitaldophilus to clear the intestinal tract, together with her gynaecologist whose expert attention cleared her infections and opened the Fallopian tubes, gave her a little 6 lb 8 oz girl who is, we are told, 'healthy, lively and very intelligent'.

High cadmium

Mr and Mrs S.L., who live on the south coast, had been infertile for some time when they got in touch with us. She was 34 years old, and like so many women of this age, regarded 35 years as 'the watershed'. Analysis revealed a very high level of cadmium in both her and her husband. (This is something we find along the south coast at times, and we would welcome comments.) They were non-smokers and we were unable to trace the source, but we cleansed this and sorted out their essential minerals, and their daughter was born weighing 8 lb 7 oz.

Combining with other infertility treatment

A midwife came to us who had been infertile for 18 months. 'I do long for one I can keep!' she told us. She followed some of the Foresight programme, but also took 'the smallest possible dose of Clomid, just once'. This combined operation brought her a lovely boy, 7 lb 5 oz. She followed the Foresight principles for her second pregnancy and, without any Clomid, she had a little girl of 6 lb 11 oz.

Another lady, who was 37 years old and did not want to wait, combined our dietary advice with 'just one small dose of Clomid', conceived straight away, and had a girl, 7 lb 3 oz.

Another midwife, however, was very determined she did NOT want to use Clomid. By clearing the toxic metals, and by supplementing zinc and other minerals, she won through and conceived her third child at age 44 years. 'I just felt the Foresight approach was so right, so logical, I knew once everything was just as it should be, I would conceive, I was never worried,' she told us. 'And I must have been right, as I was only two hours in labour!'

Another couple were waiting for a further attempt at IVF after three previous ones had failed to achieve implantation. They had been warned they might never have children, and the woman was very miserable about this. Mrs L.V. was a vegetarian, and, as is sometimes the case, had not been able to find the advice she needed to make her diet adequate. Her Foresight programme corrected her zinc deficiency and cleansed the toxic metals that had accumulated. The importance of organic produce was stressed and she started eating a much wider variety of foods, which included eggs, yoghurts and cheeses, as luckily she was not allergic to dairy produce. When the letter arrived to summon them for the next attempt at IVF Mrs L.V. was well on the way with her pregnancy and her 7 lb 15 oz daughter arrived a few months later. 'She is so healthy and she so loves life,' they wrote to us.

Miscarriage

Sometimes the problem is not one of infertility but of not being able to see the pregnancy through to term because of miscarriage(s).

We had a letter from Scotland in 1985. Mrs L. had suffered two miscarriages, then had a little son, and then suffered a further miscarriage. She was 39 years old and wanted a companion for her little boy, and she felt that time was running out. She was found to have a very high level of lead and cadmium. We see these high levels from Scotland: the acid soil from the pine and heather countryside produces very acid water, and this can wear through the old lead piping, which may then be repaired with a plug of amalgam which contains cadmium. Mr and Mrs L. were both non-smokers so this seemed the most likely explanation. We suggested a water filter and a programme of supplements. The dietary programme to cleanse toxic metals included peas, beans and lentils, Vitamin C, onions and garlic and especially the B-Complex vitamins, manganese and zinc. Funds were a problem so they used Brewer's Yeast, Vitamin C and the dietary measures. The following year their little boy was born at 7 lb 6 oz. 'He is super.'

Pre-eclampsia
Mrs M. wrote to us in 1982, after losing her first baby at 23 weeks due to pre-eclampsia. Previous to this tragedy she had suffered a miscarriage. She told us she was 39 years old so she was understandably anxious. In those days we had to send our hair samples to USA, which took a little longer. When the results were sent back, they showed a very high level of lead and some low essential minerals. In those days we were not acquainted with water filters and many of the environmental tips we can suggest now were unknown to us, but we were able to give her a cleansing programme and supplement the minerals she needed. She became pregnant again sooner than anyone expected, but this pregnancy lasted until 36 weeks when she gave birth to a tiny girl, 5 lb 3 oz. She then told us she was 41 years old when she contacted us, but had not told us before in case we thought she was too old, and advised her against the pregnancy. Her daughter, she told us, 'is beautiful, eats well, sleeps well, smiles all the time'.

Desire for better pregnancy outcomes
Mrs T.S. had also suffered PET with a previous pregnancy and her baby boy had had to be brought into the world very abruptly weighing just over 3 lb. He had survived, but his parents very much hoped that they should not have to go through the trauma of a premature birth again. The hair analysis showed the usual low essential minerals, including zinc, a high level of copper and some toxic metals. This was all duly corrected and in due course 'our' baby girl arrived, weighing 8 lb 11 oz.

Mrs O.R. wrote from the West Country, a little worried as her last baby had only weighed 5 lb 9 oz, although born at 41 weeks. A hair analysis showed very high levels of lead and aluminium, and low levels of most of the essential minerals. It took a little while, but she persevered very gamely with her programme, and when her Foresight son eventually appeared she wrote to us that he weighed 8 lb 6 oz and that she had had a home birth with the help of a midwife. 'The only problem is bright red hair!' she wrote. 'Are there any minerals that tone that down a bit?' I wrote back, 'My red-haired son has just grown a bright red beard, you ain't seen nut'ing yet!'

Mrs R.J. came to us after two unstable pregnancies, both with bleeding and pain throughout, and ending in a premature birth and a small baby (two pre-term babies). Both children had survived and were thriving, but the experience had been rather nerve-racking and she hoped for an easier pregnancy next time. She suffered from asthma and migraine. Her Foresight clinician checked for viruses and allergies, gave treatment as necessary and sorted out the minerals. Her third pregnancy sailed ahead without problems and her little boy arrived at 8 lb 4 oz and in very good order, despite a caesarian due to a breech presentation.

Mrs E.J.M. came to us, very worried at 33 years. She had had a miscarriage followed by three years of infertility and investigations on the NHS. After this, she had been happy to find she was pregnant again, only to suffer from pre-eclamptic toxaemia and lose this baby also. Like so many, when she came to us, she was not sure that she could bear to start another pregnancy. She had the Foresight supplementation and cleansing programme, but her husband was not sure he could stand the strain of another pregnancy, and for a while we heard no more. I was so pleased when three years later she got back in touch, to tell us she had had two little girls, very close in age, of 7 lb 10 oz and 7 lb 8 oz. 'They are great companions, and they have such beautiful complexions... they seem to benefit by our dietary regime and have much fewer colds than their contemporaries seem to have – all round it was lucky we found you!'

Malformations

With some babies there is the double loss, the baby was malformed and his life was lost. This makes the thought of the next pregnancy even more concerning.

Mrs J. came to us having previously given birth to two babies suffering anencephaly, both stillborn. She was a very independent lady who wanted to read all the research for herself, was interested in the books on diet and the Foresight vitamins and minerals. She changed to a wholefood diet and worked out a regime of supplements for herself. Her little girl was born, nine days late, weighing 8 lb 9 oz. She had felt confident using her own judgement, using information we could supply, and it had worked out very well.

Mrs Q. had previously had a miscarriage at 23 weeks, the baby having a malformed abdomen. She was 41 years old, and this had been a first, much wanted pregnancy. She was understandably very shattered. Despite the pressure that being over 40 years always exerts – on all of us – she very sensibly waited to complete the Foresight programme and was then rewarded by conceiving the very next month. This proved to be the redoubtable gentleman she later described to us: 'A beautiful, big, bright, bouncing boy!' (7 lb 5 oz).

A lady who has proved to be one of the most positive supporters was Mrs M.D.T. who came to us firstly after the stillbirth of a malformed baby followed by a miscarriage. She was then, as she put it, 'devastated, suffering from exhaustion, depression and from a complete dearth of any information that might help'. Her Foresight clinician soon discovered her food allergies and deficiencies and put her on a programme of supplements. She read everything we could provide and we introduced her to our favourite bookshop, 'Wholefood'. Her lovely little daughter was born at 7 lb 13½ oz, 'as fit as a fiddle', said her delighted parents. Mrs M.T.D. is now a mine of information and keeps in touch and is keeping abreast of new developments.

Hearing about a tragedy with a baby is something one can never get used to and some letters really break one's heart. Mr and Mrs V.'s first baby had been born with a malformation and had died in the womb. They had then suffered an early miscarriage. Two years later their second daughter was born with the same malformation and died after just one day. They came to us very uncertain that anything Foresight could do would help. Their doctor was dubious, and at first they did not do very much that was suggested, just altering their diet and some aspects of their lifestyle. Sadly, another miscarriage took place. This convinced them, however, that to go all the way with Foresight was the only thing worth trying. Once the decision had been made, they stuck with it, and went 100 per cent of the way with all the suggested programme. The fifth pregnancy resulted in a perfectly formed and beautiful little girl, 7 lb 14 oz. They sent one of the most touching letters we have ever received.

From the Midlands, we heard another very sad history. Mrs L.K.I. told us her first baby was stillborn with anencephaly, and this was followed very shortly by a miscarriage. Then, very fortunately, she had a little boy who was small but perfectly formed. They thought their luck had turned and she conceived again, but this fourth pregnancy ended with the birth of a baby girl with Turner's Syndrome, who died almost immediately. On contacting Foresight, hair analysis of both parents revealed a number of aberrant levels, including very high magnesium, low potassium (which can indicate allergies), low zinc and manganese and some toxic metals. After being on the Foresight programme for a few months the fifth pregnancy took us all by surprise, but in due course along came the little girl her mother described to us as 'such a pretty baby, huge eyes and perfect lips'. Later we were sent a photo of her in her christening robe – and yes, she really is a *very* pretty baby!

Heart defects
A very brave lady, Mrs S.E., had had two little boys born with heart defects. Tragically, each had died in the first few days of life, although

efforts had been made to save them. She had been put off the idea of hair analysis by medical scepticism, and she elected just to take the vitamins and minerals 'blind' and Vitamin C. Luckily this proved effective, and her third boy was born at 8 lb 14 oz and, as she said, 'very healthy and thank God, with a normal heart'.

Some years ago Mrs A. got in touch from Merseyside after her first son had been born with a heart condition. Hair samples sent to USA revealed a hugely high copper and lead level in both partners. She told us her husband spent a lot of time driving on the motorway. High copper in the wife makes one suspect the pill or the copper coil, but in this case it was stemming from the drinking water. It took nearly a year of filtered water, cleansing programmes (and help from a homeopathic doctor they were visiting who realised the significance of the metals also) to get a normal reading. Their little boy, born 7 lb 10 oz, was, they told us, 'born in perfect condition, we have never had a moment's worry with him'.

More than once we have been contacted by an anxious relative...

This was the case with Mrs C.V. Her sister wrote to us as she had just suffered a second miscarriage and was suffering from suicidal depression. We suggested big vitamin and mineral supplements with plenty of zinc. This lifted the depression enough for her to agree with her sister that she should seek help from a Foresight clinician. Discussing the probable reasons for the miscarriage and seeing the results of the various tests helped to restore her confidence. Following treatment, the next year she had an 8 lb daughter, and her sister, who had gone over to help for the first few weeks, rang me and said, 'She is the most contented baby I have ever known, and her mother is thrilled with her.'

Potential grannies are often in touch and if this is the mother-in-law, this can need tact! However, one of our happier contacts was from the mother of a daughter in Africa who had had three miscarriages. Circumstances did not permit the couple to travel home, but letters went to and fro and we were able to give some guidelines. In due course, the long awaited baby was about to arrive and her granny flew out... 'She is absolutely beautiful and I was holding her in my arms when she was 10 minutes old,' we were told. The baby weighed 7 lb 8 oz.

Allergies

Some mothers come to us because of their own problems with allergic illness. Sometimes these are very severe, as with eczema, asthma, migraine, etc, and some are taking quite a lot of potentially feto-toxic medication such as steroids, painkillers, etc.

Mrs F.N. suffered from migraine and dizzy spells and was sensitive to hydrocarbons and other inhaled allergens. She got rid of some toxic metal, improved her mineral levels and the B-Complex vitamins and Vitamins A, E and C, and had a course of desensitisation. Then she felt ready to face a pregnancy. Her son was born in hospital, 7 lb 10 oz, and they went home the same day. 'We were both very well,' she said. 'He was an alert, happy baby, right from the start.'

Cleft palate

Mrs C.L. wrote to us that she could not afford to do the Foresight programme in full, but her little boy had been born with a cleft palate and she did not want to risk this happening with a second child. We advised no smoking for both partners, as smoking is known to increase the risk of clefts, suggested she took large amounts of Vitamin C to clear any toxins, and the Foresight vitamins and minerals to provide any vitamins and trace elements that might have been missing. Animal research has linked clefts with lack of B-Complex vitamins, and epidemiology has linked it with use of pesticides which can mean shortage of choline, manganese and essential fatty acids. Her second little boy was born a week early, but with perfect facial structure.

Older mothers

Some mothers come to us just because they feel they are 'old' for this particular pregnancy. Sometimes it is the first baby, sometimes they would just like one more to complete their family.

One such was Mrs C.A. who wrote us such a cheerful letter. She had just got married, aged 42 – she had no health problems that she knew of, and saw no reason why she should not have a baby! Nor did we, and we made a speedy appointment with a Foresight clinician. As can be the way with the older ladies, the pregnancy took a little time to get under way, but Mrs C.A. stuck with the programme and remained optimistic, and just after her 44th birthday a little girl arrived weighing 7 lb 7½ oz and, her mother told us, 'very healthy, lively and beautiful!'

Some older mothers also have health problems of their own they are anxious not to pass on to the baby.

In one household the mother and two daughters suffered from asthma. We suggested various possible allergens to look out for, and moving the gas boiler to outside the house. She consulted her Foresight clinician who was also a homeopath, and minerals and diet were adjusted. Once things were easier, she felt ready for her pregnancy, and it was at age 41 years she had her son, 9 lb 9 oz. 'I was by far the oldest mother in the ward, and he was by far the biggest baby,' she told us. 'But we seemed to have the easiest time of anyone, it was quite strange really!'

Another 'older' mother wrote from the north of Scotland. She had two 'lads' but had since had two miscarriages. 'They tell me I must be mad because I am 42, but I do want another baby and it might be a little girl,' she told us. I suspected high lead might be causing the miscarriages, as we see this so often from Scotland, but no, when the charts came back this was not the case. There were just very low levels of all the vital nutrients, probably reflecting the exhaustion of looking after two lively 'laddies' and having the two miscarriages. It took about a year to get things right, but she persevered, and in due course along came another little boy – which is what his brothers had been hoping for! He weighed in at 8 lb 10 oz, and is, his mother says, 'a wonderful, peaceful, contented baby, just right for elderly parents'.

A lovely Jewish lady rang me, very frustrated. She had five beautiful daughters, of whom she was immensely proud, but it was very important to her husband to have a son. She was 43 years old, very willing to have another pregnancy but she had developed fibroids and her gynaecologist thought it unlikely she would conceive again. She flourished under one of our most experienced clinicians, and her copper levels were reduced and her zinc levels restored to normal. (Zinc is important to the male fetus.) The pregnancy progressed for 36 weeks and then the welcome son put in his appearance, weighing 5 lb 15 oz. 'He is such a jolly little boy,' says his mother. One would expect he has plenty to be jolly about!

Mrs V.W. was a strict vegetarian and was suffering from a virus, anaemia and 'constant fatigue'. Her Foresight doctor sorted out the infection and got her to wait to start her pregnancy until her diet was much improved and her mineral levels were good. She has since had two splendid little boys of 8 lb 7 oz and 9 lb 3 oz.

Mrs D.W. wrote from the north. She had, she told us, 'lots of allergies which produce asthma and eczema, so I have to stick to a very restricted diet'. Her doctor was very friendly and interested in all that we found, and he encouraged her to supplement her deficiencies. Her two little Foresight boys (7 lb 5 oz and 7 lb 15 oz) have so far remained clear of all allergic reactions, except to one food. She tells us they are 'wonderfully healthy little boys'.

Tranquilliser addiction
Another mother, Mrs J.I., wrote to us very distressed because she found she was addicted to the tranquillisers which had been given to her to help her get over two former miscarriages. She did not want to risk a pregnancy while taking them, so they were compounding the problem. She had quite a fight to get off them, but was helped by her Foresight clinician and the supplements – magnesium, manganese and iron all had been very low, and these are helpful in depression – and in the end she won through. Quite soon after this we heard that she was pregnant, and in due course the little girl arrived at 6 lb 11 oz. 'A very happy girl,' says her mother.

Club feet
Some parents come to us because of malformations in the family, or because they have suffered one themselves.

One mother contacted us from the north of Scotland because she had been born with club feet. She was a very bright, communicative lady, very interested in all the research, and in doing all she could. In due course her son was born, with perfect feet, 'So strong and healthy,' she told us (6 lb 15 oz).

Mrs G.F.D. was one of the many mothers who have become a great friend through many telephone calls. She first came to me aged 39 years. She and her husband had been married for 12 years, but had just decided it was time to have a child. She was willing to see a Foresight clinician and have the mineral analyses, but he was very sceptical. She started to prepare for the pregnancy and then there was a change of plan. His work was to take them to Canada and she decided that, at nearly 40 years of age, she was too old to be travelling around the globe, moving house and pregnant! We wished them every happiness and off they went. Two years later they were back in England regretting this decision. They had been living with relatives with a large happy family and they felt they had missed out. They were hoping they could still achieve a child. She was then aged 42 years, but this time her husband decided he would join in, so we quickly got an appointment for them and things got under way. Minerals were not too bad and soon pregnancy took place and along came her little boy, 7 lb 6 oz. 'All my friends told me it would be tough going at my age, and it would be tiring – some of them tried to make me reconsider,' she wrote. 'Nobody told me how much fun he would be and how much we would love him.' She has no regrets.

Eczema
Many mothers seek our help because of allergic or other health problems in a previous child.

Mrs W.E. came to us about her second pregnancy, her first child having suffered milk allergy with diarrhoea and failed to thrive. She was also much troubled with eczema. This baby had been conceived with a copper IUD in place, and during the pregnancy the mother had suffered high blood pressure. When she came to us, two years later, her hair analysis still showed the high copper, typical of Copper 7 IUD users. She also had other high toxic metals. The levels were restored to normal and the Foresight pregnancy went ahead without a hitch and her little girl was born full-term, 8 lb ½ oz.

Late starters
Some mothers start on the Foresight regime late in the pregnancy as they have not heard of us until the pregnancy is well under way. We try to do all we can – although we much prefer to start at the beginning!

Mrs M.O.'s first son had allergies, asthma and eczema almost from birth, and this and the broken nights with the bottle-feeding and his crying during the day, coupled with her own exhaustion, gave her post-partum depression for over a year. Her family all begged her not to risk another pregnancy, but she had not wanted her little boy to be an only child. 'He got off to a very bad start, and I felt this would just be another deprivation,' she told us. We advised on diet and supplements. We also helped to clear the very high level of lead and supplement the low zinc in her little boy that was causing the aberrant behaviour. She also filtered the water to guard against toxic metals. She rang in from the hospital when her second little boy (7 lb 14 oz) was six hours old. 'I feel better six hours after this birth than I did six months after the last one,' she told us. This little boy was fully breastfed and weighed 11 lb 14 oz at seven weeks – and no eczema. 'My mother can't thank you enough,' she wrote to us. 'She is just utterly amazed how much difference those little tablets can make – she thought it was just me!'

Amniocentesis

Some years ago a lovely Italian lady rang me, very upset. She was 44 years old and pregnant with her seventh, much wanted child. The hospital was pressing her re amniocentesis, because of her age and the risk of Down's syndrome. She was frightened to submit to the test in case she lost the baby. Down's syndrome has been associated with low levels of selenium in American research papers. I suggested I sent her the papers, and we sent hair to the lab. The chart came back with an excellent level of selenium. We discussed this, in the light of what was known, and the excellent provisions for Down's syndrome children, and she decided to bypass the test. In due course her seventh son arrived in very good order at 7 lb 15 oz. Now at nursery school, there are problems! 'They say he is so cheeky to all the teachers, even the headmaster! I had to go round ...But I say, you must let me explain the situation. One of his brothers is an international lawyer, one is in the Diplomatic Service, one is a doctor...He is used to treating them as his contemporaries...'

PART TWO

The need for intervention

CHAPTER 3

Preconception Care

WHY YOU ARE RIGHT TO BE SEEKING HELP *BEFORE* YOU START YOUR PREGNANCY.

And the angel of the Lord appeared unto the woman, and said unto her, 'Behold now thou art barren, and bearest not: but thou shalt conceive, and bear a son.
'Now therefore beware, I pray thee, and drink not wine nor strong drink, and eat not any unclean thing.[1]

An old practice

Preconception care is not a new concept. Not only can advice be found in the Bible, it abounds in the many traditions passed down through generations, and sometimes relegated to the status of 'old wives' tales'. It knows no boundaries – Dr Weston Price (see page 52) found that many tribes across the world had preconception programmes which paid particular attention to nutrition. In the Masai tribe, this planning even extended to the time a girl was allowed to marry. This had to be after she had had a few months on a diet which included milk from cows which had been grazed on rapidly growing young grass. This was known to be very nutritious. In other parts of the world fish, and especially fish eggs, were highly prized in the preconception period. Sometimes preparation was extended to the father-to-be as well.[2]

Work on animals confirmed the wisdom of these practices. It is widely acknowledged in zoos today that if animals are to breed successfully (wild animals are scarce!) they need optimal care and this includes the right nutrition.[3]

In this book, we are not attempting to convince you that you should consider a new practice – we are seeking to pass on wisdom which has been part of world culture for centuries, only now we can understand the rationale for it. We are also presenting research into new dangers faced by prospective parents, dangers which are of our own making.

The necessity for preconception care

But some of you will be saying that Britain's children are healthier than they have ever been, with less deformity, fewer stillbirths and perinatal deaths. Our women do not die in childbirth. Antenatal care is available to any woman who seeks it. Do we actually need to consider preconception care?

The answer to this question was provided by Dr Hamish Sutherland of the Department of Obstetrics of Gynaecology, University of Aberdeen, in a letter to *The Lancet* in 1982 in which he said:

> Too many women make (their) first antenatal visit with the pregnancy already compromised or at risk from smoking, inappropriate nutrition, ingestion of a variety pharmaceutical preparations (including oral contraceptive steroids), genito-urinary infection, anaemia, and poor dental hygiene. All too frequently cervical cytology and rubella immunity status are unknown.[4]

We may have the means to have better food (though we often choose to ignore them) and most of us have better living conditions than our grandparents, but we have also added a new range of dangers to the fetus and child, some of which Sutherland has mentioned. Others include increasing air and water pollution, and increasing radiation from both non-ionising and ionising sources (see pages 109–111). Chemicals in the workplace can be especially hazardous. The result is that we still have more adverse pregnancy outcomes than is necessary, given the state of our knowledge.

The extent of the problems

Although reports in recent years have shown that there are variations between regions and classes, we shall concentrate on the British national figures. Suffice to say that the lower the income and the further north, the greater is the risk of poor health generally, including fetal and child health.[5]

Poor pregnancy outcomes which are recorded (and many are not, including such conditions as epilepsy and dyslexia) fall into a number of categories. Those which end in death are categorised according to the time of death. The Office of Population Censuses and Surveys (OPCS) draws the following distinctions:

28 complete weeks of gestation to birth – stillbirth.
Stillbirths and deaths in first week of life – perinatal death.
Birth to 28 days of life – neonatal death.
Death when over 28 days but under one year of age – post-neonatal death.
Death at aged under one year – infant death.

Overall the trend in all categories has been downward. For example, in 1980 we had a perinatal mortality rate of 13.3 per 1,000 total births (England and Wales): by 1986 it was 9.6.[6] But we should not be complacent. The Foresight experience and the various research data we present in this book lead to the conclusion that we could reduce still further these figures. If we consider the international situation, we may have improved but other nations have done even better so our overall ranking has not changed much, as shown in the table overleaf.

Infant mortality rates for selected countries – 1975 and 1983.[7]
(Rates per 100,000 total live births.)

Rank (1975)	Country	1975	Rank (1983)	1983
1	Sweden	859.8	3	702.8
2	Japan	1004.7	2	623.5
3	Denmark	1032.3	5	771.3
4	Netherlands	1064.8	7	841.1
5	Switzerland	1074.4	4	760.3
6	Finland	1102.9	1	612.9
7	Norway	1109.2	6	791.0
8	France	1380.0	8	913.0
9	Australia	1427.0	9	959.3
10	**England and Wales**	**1572.3**	10	**1014.3**
11	New Zealand	1601.4	12	1285.8
12	USA	1606.9	11	1124.2

This places us with a rate that is over 60 per cent greater than Finland, the country in the top rank. In 1984, England and Wales had an infant mortality rate 61 per cent greater than Sweden.[8]

If we go further back in time the situation was similar. Between 1955 and 1972 we changed from ranking 13 to 11 in a list of 15 selected countries, including all those listed above, in respect of perinatal deaths. As Dr Lambert wrote, when he published the figures, 'With a rate that is 50 per cent greater than the lowest (Sweden) there is clearly room for improvement'.[9]

The situation in the Netherlands is of particular interest, since they have a different approach to birth, with most deliveries done by midwives, and only five per cent of births not being completely natural, without drugs and other intervention. Most of the improvement in the other countries is attributed to improved antenatal and postnatal care. However, we should not overlook the facts that the Scandinavian countries generally have more stringent food additive policies, a better standard of nutrition, and are more pollution conscious. Other countries with better figures than ours also tend to have a lower proportion of low birth weight babies (see below) and congenital deformities.[10]

Turning to congenital malformations we see another disappointing picture, though there has been considerable change in the figures since the introduction of screening and abortion. (But the figures do not show the pain suffered by those couples who decide on an abortion.) The rates, per 10,000 live births, have decreased from 215.8 in 1977 to 197.1 in 1986. But there were still 13,097 babies born with congenital malformations, including 12,758 live births. Central nervous system malformations continue to decline, due mainly to a large fall in the incidence of spina bifida. (See Chapter 5.) The rate for this condition in 1977 was 15.3: in 1986 it was 4.0. But it is likely that improved nutrition could reduce this figure still further! Ear malformations and cardiovascular problems have slightly increased over the last ten years.[11]

It is difficult to assess many other problems associated with reproduction and its successful outcome. We do not know how many couples are involuntarily infertile, partly because the definition of 'infertility' differs among researchers, though we do know that there has been an 'astonishing' increase in the last generation.[12] We do know that the demand for special education is increasing as more children have learning difficulties. We do know that there is an increase in anti-social behaviour among children. We do know that there is an increase in mental illness. We suspect that not all the increase in child abuse cases is due to better reporting. All the factors point to a lack of success in reproductive outcome. But how can problems arise? Before answering this, let us look briefly at some of the steps in the actual process of reproduction.

The process of reproduction

Reproduction is not a simple process – there are many steps involved, each with its own pitfalls, but we do know from animals and human research that healthy reproduction is not difficult if both partners are in the peak of health. (See Chapters 2–14.)

Starting with the boy, he begins his preparation for fatherhood in his mother's womb, when his organs are developing. He continues it throughout his childhood. In this process, indeed throughout life, excellent nutrition is needed for maximum effect. At puberty he starts producing sperm in his testes. At the appropriate time, the sperm pass down tubules where they are ejaculated from the penis into the woman's vagina in a liquid called semen, which is produced by the seminal vesicles and prostate glands.

Of the millions of sperm deposited in the vagina less than 100 ever reach the egg in the Fallopian tube and even they have to wait for a few hours until they are capable of fertilising it. This ability is associated with increased motility. (See below)

Like the boy, the girl's preparations begin in the womb, when her eggs are developed. During this period the fetal ovaries contain up to 6.8 million oocytes, although these decrease to around 2 million at birth and 60,000 at puberty. If the mother is not healthy, she could be laying the foundation for problems in her subsequent grandchildren, or even causing infertility in her daughter. At puberty the girl starts to menstruate, having cycles of fertility and infertility. (See Chapter 6.) If she is to reproduce successfully she will need to ensure that her reproductive organs are healthy. Her Fallopian tubes need to be clear of obstructions and infections so the egg can pass down with ease. Her womb lining needs to be healthy for implantation. Her vagina and cervix need to be free from infection both for the sperm and the baby during its birth. Once the egg is implanted she needs to provide good nutrition for it to develop, and a healthy environment, free from toxins.

When fertilisation has taken place, it will take three or four days for the fertilised egg to reach the womb and a further three days for it to be implanted. By now the cells in it will have been dividing continually since fertilisation, each reproducing Deoxyribose Nucleic Acid (DNA). This process of growth and division will continue throughout life. Sometimes the DNA will not be perfectly reproduced but will correct itself later on. It is only when such correction is not made that there are difficulties such as deformity.

Both the production of sperm and of the egg are controlled by hormones in the body, which is why any condition affecting the endocrine system can have adverse consequences for fertility.

The developing embryo grows very quickly, so that by eight weeks in gestation the limbs can be seen quite easily. As Sutherland said (see above), by then it can be too late to consider preventive measures. This is why Foresight has paid particular attention to the period before conception.

What can go wrong?

In this section we shall look at both fertility and pregnancy outcome for both partners, though this is but a brief survey. We start with the male to stress his importance in the process and final outcome, since it is often overlooked that he is responsible, either fully or in part, for between 30 and 50 per cent of infertility, the actual figure varying according to the authority being quoted. No one has assessed his likely part in problem pregnancies, though it is likely to be significant if his sperm is not healthy.

The main reasons for infertility and fertility problems in the man include:

1 Absence of live sperm in the semen. This can arise because of structural problems, such as blocked or twisted tubes, or no tubes at all. In Klinefelter's syndrome there is actual sterility. The endocrine system may not be working properly to stimulate the production of sperm. (Of course, if a vasectomy has been performed in the past this will also block the passage of the sperm to the semen!)

2 Scarcity of sperm in the semen – low sperm count. This can arise where the testes have failed to descend outside the body. Drug therapy for tumours, infertility or low sperm count may also cause problems. Other medical conditions, such as varicocele, can lower the count: Vitamin E is needed for healthy veins, so nutritional imbalances may be a factor. Certain chemicals in the workplace, as well as social drugs, can have similar effects. (See Chapters 8 and 10.) Generally speaking, it is reckoned that a man has a low count if he has less than 20 million sperm in a millilitre of semen. One researcher has shown that 23 per cent of male students at Florida State University have sperm counts that are functionally sterile, that is lower than 20 million sperm per millilitre of semen, a result similar to the 20 per cent in other studies. This compares with 0.5 per cent in 1938.[13]

3 Impaired sperm function. The sperm may have poor motility and

fail to reach the egg. They do, after all, have to travel a long way! The sperm then has actually to penetrate the egg, which it may fail to do, especially if there is a lack of zinc. Infection with chlamydia, for example, will also affect sperm function, as will social drugs. (See Chapters 8 and 9.)

4 Unhealthy sperm. If the sperm is not healthy when it fertilises the egg, assuming it is able to, the fetus may not develop normally. It is now known, for example, that either the man or woman may be responsible for a Down's syndrome baby.[14] Social drugs, especially alcohol and nicotine, will cause adverse effects.

In the woman, there may be problems associated with:

1 Ovulation. The endocrine system may not be working properly to release the necessary hormones. Disease, severe nutritional disturbances, allergies, malabsorption, significant weight loss, strenuous physical activity, stress, exposure to chemical and physical agents, such as the pill or radiation, can also interfere with ovulation.
2 Structural faults. These may be congenital, with perhaps a lack of organs, or faulty organs. This may include blocked or twisted Fallopian tubes, though these are often the result of infections, zinc deficiency or oedema. (See Chapters 8 and 13.) Previous sterilisation may be a factor. This will stop the egg from reaching the sperm. The environment in the vagina, uterus and tubes may not be healthy enough to support the sperm through its journey. The womb lining may not be healthy enough for implantation.
3 Medical conditions such as endometriosis, polyps, and/or fibroids, or pelvic inflammatory disease can affect fertility and, in some cases, pregnancy outcome. (See Chapter 13.)
4 Age decreases fertility, though some research suggests that 'under ideal conditions the effect of age on the chance of achieving a successful pregnancy may be less than previous studies have led us to believe'.[15] Certainly, women over the age of 40 years can have successful pregnancy outcomes with the correct preparation, as the Foresight experience has shown. (See Chapter 2.)
5 The egg may not be healthy and may be incapable of developing after fertilisation. Alternatively, it may develop but produce abnormalities. It may also implant while still in the Fallopian tube, causing an ectopic pregnancy.
6 If the egg is implanted, the woman may not be healthy enough to maintain the pregnancy, perhaps because of poor nutritional status, infections, allergic illness or the presence of toxins. (See Chapters 5, 7, 8, 10 and 13.) Alternatively, she may maintain the pregnancy but the outcome may not be satisfactory.
7 If the birth is completed, there may be subsequent problems, such as with lactation and future development of the baby.

Problems of pregnancy outcome

Assuming a pregnancy has occurred there are a number of possible outcomes. We believe that, with the correct preconception care, in most cases the outcome should be a healthy baby, with healthy parents to guide its future development into a healthy adult, able, in turn, to reproduce healthy offspring.

However, there are alternative results which are not happy. We have already discussed the incidence of stillbirth, congenital malformations and neonatal deaths. Other major problems include miscarriage, preterm babies, low birth weight, developmental disabilities, behavioural disorders, chronic diseases, malignancies, intrauterine growth retardation and chromosomal abnormalities. Let us look in more detail at some of the problems.

Infertility

Infertility is generally reckoned to be present when a couple has failed to start a pregnancy within a year of trying. Although we said earlier that we did not know how many couples were infertile there have been a number of studies which suggest figures of about one in ten[16] or one in eight, with one in six couples seeking help with a first or subsequent pregnancy.[17] There are many causes, as we have already indicated, and we would not claim that the Foresight approach will relieve all infertility, though it can help quite a large number of couples because it tackles many of the factors which lead to infertility, especially biochemical imbalances and disease. Sadly, there will be those, for example, whose tubes are so damaged that pregnancy through sexual intercourse is impossible. In vitro fertilisation (IVF) or the use of donated sperm (AID) may be alternatives, though the latter does have many more psychological problems for both partners, which are frequently overlooked.[18] However, the Foresight programme will still be relevant in becoming healthy for the pregnancy. IVF has a high failure rate, and it is our experience that success is more likely if both partners are healthy.

Miscarriage – or spontaneous abortion

Some miscarriages occur very early in the pregnancy, so the woman may not even have realised she was pregnant. For miscarriage occurring later on, the incidence may be about 15 per cent, but there are no reliable studies. Some say that one in four of women who become pregnant will have one or more miscarriages.[19] Women who tend to have repeat miscarriages are more likely to have chromosomally normal aborted fetuses, so it seems likely that the fault lies in the mother's ability to carry the fetus. This suggests that her health is of great importance. It has been questioned if a slow-down in the synthesis of DNA is a factor in early miscarriage, since a deficiency of many nutrients can slow it down, as well as causing chromosomal damage.[20] Yet again, we must stress that good nutrition seems crucial. The research findings we present in chapter 5 show that deficiencies in a number of nutrients are associated with low birth weight, including essential fatty acids, Vitamin B1, calcium, copper, cobalt, magnesium and zinc. But many other factors may be involved, including radiation, drugs, smoking, chemicals and physical hazards at home and in the workplace, infections and diseases.

The Foresight experience so far suggests that the rate of miscarriage can be drastically reduced if the Foresight programme is followed.

Preterm babies

There is sometimes confusion over the terms 'preterm' and 'prematurity'. Preterm babies include those born early, before full term, who were previously known as premature babies, and those babies who weigh less than 5 lb 8 oz at birth. In some medical papers, prematurity is still the word used for early births.

The causes for babies born with a short gestation period, i.e. approximately 28 to 34 weeks after conception instead of 40 weeks, are many, including:

- Malnutrition.
- Inadequate prenatal care.
- Unfortunate socio-economic conditions.
- Multiple pregnancies where the uterus walls cannot expand anymore.
- Excessive smoking.
- Oxygen starvation.
- Emotional disturbances (which probably affect nutritional status).
- Drugs.
- Some illnesses, e.g. syphilis.
- Age: especially where a young woman has had a succession of babies.
- First baby after the age of 40 years.
- Complications in pregnancy, e.g. infections, toxaemia.[21]
- Heavy metal toxicity.[22]
- Births induced too early because of confusion over dates.
- Zinc/copper imbalances caused by the pill or copper IUD.[23]
- All sexually transmitted diseases, which appear to have adverse effects according to the experiences of Foresight clinicians.

Studies quote demographic factors, such as socioeconomic status, age, marital status and education. In our experience, these are not reasons in themselves; most can be linked with the mother's health status before and during pregnancy, especially the existence of infection, her nutritional status, her history of substance abuse and exposure to toxins such as heavy metals and drugs. Low socioeconomic status may be the result of a poor educational status, and may mean low pay, with little money being spent on good food, assuming she is educated about the importance of healthy eating.

Preterm babies may suffer from a range of physical, psychological and intellectual problems. They have a wrinkled look and may be too weak to suck. Their brain may be too immature to control breathing or body temperature. They are prone to infection as their immune system is immature.[24]

Babies who weigh less than 5 lb 8 oz (2,500 grams) at birth are said to have a low birth weight. If they are under 3 lb 5 oz (1,500 grams) they are of very low birth weight. Those with a birth weight between 4 lb 6½ oz and 5 lb 8 oz (2,000–2,500 grams) will tend to have only slight problems which are overcome with time. However, for those under 4 lb 6½ oz (2,000 grams) the outlook is poorer, and they are likely to have some type of developmental difficulty.[25] The causes include those mentioned above. Prenatal malnutrition is undoubtedly a major damaging factor in low birth weight, as famine studies have shown,[26] though smoking more than 20 cigarettes a day doubles the risk.[27] Other factors include malformation of the uterus, fibroid tumours, high blood pressure, and genetic causes, such as maternal and paternal size, poor weight gain, poor obstetric history, stress and preterm labour.[28] Prolonged standing at work may also be a contributory factor.[29] But it is probably inaccurate to regard many of these as reasons for low birth weight. As in our discussion on demographic factors above, it is likely that these factors are caused by certain basic conditions, most of which overlooked in the research, including high toxic metals, biochemical imbalances and sexually transmitted diseases.

Low birth weight babies represent 6–9 per cent of all births. About 2 per cent are born suffering from intrauterine growth retardation, in which the infant's weight is well below the expected weight for gestational age, with about 7 per cent being premature. However, low birth weight is said to be the most important cause of perinatal death (about 70 per cent).[30] There is an increased risk of illness. It is associated with neurodevelopmental handicaps, congenital abnormalities, and may be a factor in lower respiratory tract infections, learning difficulties and behavioural problems.[31] Such babies may experience poorer development and health because their fragility may make their parents afraid to handle them and all babies need the stimulation of touch.[32] With better neonatal care, survival rates have improved, but this does not lessen the tragedy for many parents who lose their babies or the suffering of those whose infants need medical intervention.

Health problems

Any child who is born with a medical problem, or who subsequently develops one as a result of prenatal/postnatal circumstances, is not just a statistic but the centre of a tragedy. Despite the supposedly better health care, child ill health is increasing, especially heart disease allergies, which are debilitating and sometimes life-threatening, and disorders such as hyperactivity, epilepsy and dyslexia. Yet the medical literature abounds in studies which show that the health status of both parents influences subsequent child health. (See Chapters 4–14.) After birth the environment, including pollutants and nutrition, can also affect health and development.

Conclusion

There can be no doubt that there is a need for preconception care when one examines the statistics on problem pregnancy outcomes. The Foresight approach is based on the many research findings which have been the subject of scientific study. However, in keeping with every other area of medicine, some of the work has not been tested using a scientific method. It is not easy to do some of the research ethically (see Chapter 5), nor is it always the most appropriate method. Most research ignores the fact that every subject starts at a different baseline, since we are all biochemically different. (See Chapter 5.) It denies the multifactorial nature of health problems. Many major medical approaches, including psychoanalysis and psychotherapy, have never been given rigorous testing. Any good doctor will rely on his clinical judgement if there is a discrepancy between that and laboratory findings.

Research is costly, and crossover double-blind studies are limited in their applications in the fields of reproductive and behavioural toxicology (a recent area of research which examines how poisons can affect behaviour). Until recently, it was assumed that the placenta acted as a barrier against toxins: now we know it does not. Until recently, it was assumed that the blood–brain barrier only allowed selected substances to pass – we now know that it is not as selective as we thought, especially in the fetus and young child. Cross-over studies do not allow us to assess subtle or long-term effects – for this, we need longitudinal studies and these are difficult in animals, let alone in humans. However, we now know that prenatal exposure may not reveal its damage for many years.[33] Thus a child may look normal and seem to develop normally until it is required to perform tasks which demand sophisticated perceptual processing. If some unseen damage has occurred, only then may he/she experience difficulties which interfere with learning, such as dyslexia, or behaviour, such as hyperactivity.

With the problems facing society today, including increasing national health and educational costs, there is no doubt that preconception preparation could make a contribution in saving resources.

PART THREE

Positive steps for healthy offspring

CHAPTER 4

The Preconception Medical Check – The Foresight Way

WHAT TO EXPECT IN THE WAY OF HELP AND INFORMATION FROM A PRECONCEPTUAL CHECK-UP.

If you are seeking the best opportunity for your baby to have a healthy start in life, your own health status is important. Thus, your preconception medical care is crucial.[1,2] In this chapter we outline the sort of checks the experiences of Foresight clinicians have shown need to be considered. (If your doctor is not sure of their relevance, Foresight doctors will be pleased to discuss this with him/her.) Please remember that the information given applies to both of you, though clearly some of the tests apply to only one sex.

The actual tests you have will depend on a number of factors, including your previous family and personal medical history, your present health status, your present life-style, the availability of the tests in your area, and your own wishes. First, however, let us look at the timing of intervention – when should you start your preparation?

The timing of intervention

Ideally, preparation for pregnancy should have begun during an individual's own conception, since it is then that the eggs are formed in the ovaries and healthy reproductive tracts are formed. However, we live in a less than ideal world so our planning must be over a shorter time span. Fortunately, the considerable research, some of which is cited in this book, suggests that even short-term planning is beneficial in all but a very few cases.

In an excellent review of factors involved in problem pregnancy, Arthur and Margaret Wynn have highlighted the necessity for prepregnancy planning, drawing heavily on studies of famines.[3] These have shown that congenital deformities occur in babies conceived throughout the famine, when one would expect that poor maternal nutrition is a major contributory factor, and for four months or so after the food shortage has finished. While poor nutrition may still be the cause, another factor may be damage to the germ cells (eggs or sperm) in either or both parents. Radiation which affects the male germ cells has been linked with later congenital defects. If the female germ cells in animals are irradiated on the day before conception there is a much greater incidence of chromosomal aberrations. Women who have taken medicinal drugs in the three weeks preceding conception have been found to have a higher risk of chromosomal aberrations.

The Wynns explain that it would seem that the male needs longer to recover from exposure to mutagenic substances than the female, and disagree with the recommendation of the International Commission for the Protection against Environmental Mutagens and Carcinogens (ICPEMC), which is three months. By combining all the data known they suggest a minimum of four months: 'The information from the Dutch Hunger Winter suggests that the whole legacy of disease, like childhood cancer and congenital malformations, that may have been caused by new mutations, originated mainly during the four months before conception and particularly during the four weeks before conception.'[4] Where the man is unwilling to go through the full Foresight programme (and sadly this happens) even 48 hours away from mutagens can help – though a week would be better and a month better still.[5]

The Foresight suggestion is that you seek advice six months before you plan your conception as this will allow the four months recommended by the Wynns and time for tests to be made and results to be discussed. Clearly, the timing may then need to be revised, depending on the results.

General investigation and advice

A competent doctor will take detailed histories to obtain a general picture of your health. He should ask about your family history and it is helpful to draw up a chart, like a family tree, marking against each member, known illnesses, allergies, and reasons for death. Try to cover at least as far back as your grandparents.[6] Of special interest to the doctor will be any miscarriages or abnormalities such as Down's syndrome or spina bifida.

You should be asked about your life-style, including questions about your work (see Chapter 10) and hobbies, as environmental factors related to these may have adverse effects on pregnancy. Any factors which are particularly stressful should be discussed, as stress affects health, especially nutritional status.

It is important not to become pregnant until you know you are both healthy. You should be given advice about safe methods of contraception. If you have been using the pill or coil, you should not try for a baby until your mineral levels are normal. (See Chapters 6 and 9.)

Your eating habits should be reviewed and dietary advice given. Any supplements will be prescribed when the results of your tests are through.

Smoking, alcohol and drugs are dangerous and the competent doctor will advise you accordingly. Where you are taking drugs for medical reasons, such as diabetes, eczema, asthma, migraine and/or epilepsy, alternative approaches should be considered, in order to minimise or eliminate drug-taking before and during pregnancy. Research has shown that most of these conditions respond to dietary intervention. (See Chapter 12.) Any allergies to foods, chemicals, or inhalants should be treated, possibly through desensitisation techniques. Often it will only be necessary to avoid the offending food or substance or to supplement a deficiency. Chronic infections, such as genito-urinary, ENT, respiratory and gastric, should be cleared. Some will respond to dietary methods, without needing drug treatment.

The following tests may be done:

○ BLOOD PRESSURE. This is a standard test which measures the pressure at which the heart is pumping blood round your body. High blood pressure (hypertension) can indicate a number of health conditions. Your doctor may treat you to lower it, as it could mean difficulties later on, such as pre-eclampsia in pregnancy. It is likely that this will also respond to dietary measures. (See Chapter 12.)

○ BLOOD EXAMINATION. A blood test can provide a check for zinc, copper and lead levels. (See Chapters 5 and 7.) Depending on your history, the sample may be used for checks on venereal disease (see Chapter 13), abnormalities of thyroid function (see below), Vitamin B6 deficiency (see Chapter 5), abnormalities of red and white blood cells, for conditions such as sickle cell disease and thalassaemia, both forms of anaemia, an eosinophil count to indicate an active allergy (see Chapter 12), and haemoglobin level to check for other types of anaemia. He can also test for rubella immunity (see below).

○ RUBELLA STATUS (woman only). Most people are now aware that rubella (or German measles) during pregnancy can result in a handicapped baby. (See Chapter 13.) The best prevention is vaccination before becoming pregnant, hence the ongoing vaccination programme for schoolgirls. The doctor should check your blood sample for antibodies. If the number is low, or non-existent, you should be advised to have a vaccination. You should not become pregnant for at least three months following this injection. (See Chapter 6.)

○ BASAL TEMPERATURE. This is thought to be a reliable way of testing your thyroid function. The thyroid plays an important role in the body, producing thyroxine, a hormone which has a stimulating effect on the sex hormones and sex glands. If your thyroid is underactive, there will be insufficient sex hormone output.[7]

The test involves placing a thermometer under the arm for ten minutes every morning immediately on waking (and before that early morning cuppa!). This should be done for two months, so that two menstrual cycles are checked. If the temperature is low for the whole of the cycle, your doctor should consider a thyroid function test. (See Chapters 5 and 11.)

○ URINE ANALYSIS. With a sample of your urine, the doctor can check for protein and sugar. If protein is present, it may mean that your kidneys are not working properly. (See Chapter 7.) If sugar is found it may mean the presence of diabetes. In either case, the doctor will need to do further tests. Clearly, diabetes or kidney problems are already causing stress for the woman suffering from them; pregnancy would add to the strain.

If indicated by the history, the doctor may also check for kidney infection, since this is a serious condition in pregnancy.

○ GYNAECOLOGICAL EXAMINATION (woman). This should include a smear test to check for cancer of the cervix. The doctor should also check for a prolapse, vaginal infections (preferably by a colposcope), cervical damage and pelvic abnormalities. (See Chapter 13.) Further tests may be done if the history suggests problems.

○ GENITO-URINARY EXAMINATION (man). If there is any problem with fertility, or if his partner has a history of miscarriage or infection, the doctor should do a full genito-urinary examination, especially for infection. (See Chapter 13.)

○ SEMEN SAMPLES (man). In cases of possible infertility, where you have been trying to have a baby for some time without success, the doctor should also have an up-to-date semen analysis report. He/she should also ask for one if there is any reason to suspect that the sperm could be abnormal, as in cases with a recent history of chronic ill health, coeliac condition, alcoholism, debilitating illness, surgery, or heavy smoking. (See Chapters 3, 5, 8, 12 and 13.)

○ STOOL SAMPLES. Where indicated by the history or where your hair analysis shows low levels of minerals, these can be checked for malabsorption and/or worm infestation. Anything which can interfere with the ingestion of nutrients can have serious repercussions for fertility and pregnancy outcome. (See Chapters 3 and 5.)

○ SWEAT TEST. This is a test for mineral levels which is said to be a very reliable indicator of zinc status. (See Chapter 5.) At the time of writing (May 1989), it is only available at one commercial laboratory in London and you must visit the laboratory in person (see Appendix One for address). Your doctor may advise it if there is any doubt about your mineral status, especially zinc.

○ HAIR MINERAL ANALYSIS (HMA). This test analyses the level of minerals in the hair. A sample of hair is taken from the scalp and is analysed using very sophisticated spectroscopy equipment in a medical laboratory. With these modern techniques it is possible to assess with great accuracy the level of minerals down to 0.1 parts per million or less. This is very useful as some minerals are only found in small amounts in the hair, reflecting small amounts throughout the body, although they play a vital role in life.

There have been some adverse reports on hair analysis in the media[8,9] which have been quite misleading as they have not explained how the analysis was done. In each case quoted the hair was not analysed using spectroscopy but by dowsing (using a pendulum). There have been no reliable tests using this method and it has never been recommended by Foresight.

Hair has a number of advantages over other tissues.[10-15] It is not very convenient to take samples of organ tissues, such as liver, as this requires a biopsy! Urine only tells you what the body is excreting, while blood can only show what is in it at the time the sample is taken. Most minerals are kept at near-optimum levels in the blood by a homeostatic mechanism, therefore minor deficiencies are not detectable at an early stage through blood samples. Many of the toxins, for example, are passed out of the blood very quickly. Thus, blood does not always show what is in the body. However, hair grows slowly and a properly taken sample can give a history of what has been passed into the hair follicle in the previous six to eight weeks. Moreover, it contains high levels of many minerals, often 200 times greater than in the blood. Samples can easily be taken, sent in an envelope, and stored without special arrangements. There is no risk of infection and, compared with many other tests, it is quite inexpensive. Hair mineral analysis is a useful screening tool and, especially when done in combination with blood and sweat, it gives a picture of what is happening in the body, that is adequate for clinical purposes as a guide to mineral status.

Even used on its own, it still can provide a good survey of what is going on in the body, if it is interpreted by an expert who knows what part is played by the minerals in health. Indeed, there are said to be over 1,500 citations in the scientific and medical literature confirming its usefulness.[16] The experts who use it continually are convinced that it is a valid medical test. (It is also widely used in forensic work.[17])

It is true to say that the accuracy of the test is only limited by the technician. The oft-quoted study purporting to prove it is unreliable was so poor it should never have been printed, let alone in a major medical journal![18] The researcher, Dr Barrett, claimed to have shown that 'The reported levels of most minerals varied considerably between identical samples sent to the same laboratory'.[19] However, in an excellent critique, Dr Schoenthaler has pointed out that the study was poorly designed and statistically incorrect.[20] For example, the researchers took incorrect samples of hair without telling the laboratories, and ignored the fact that the laboratories had derived their norms according to criteria that pertained to more stringent sampling methods. In a re-analysis of the data, Schoenthaler shows that there was a very high degree of reliability (96 per cent) between five of the laboratories, and an average of 92 per cent between the 'best' seven. In fact, when more meticulously examined, Barrett's data proved the opposite of what he was claiming!

Foresight and HMA
In its edition dated 9 November 1985, the *Lancet* published an editorial in which it criticised the Foresight approach, and especially its use of hair mineral analysis.[21] It is an excellent example of misguided comment, since it based its arguments on the Barrett research.

Foresight has longer experience of interpreting the hair test than any other organisation in Britain. With the enormous amount of data which shows the importance of mineral status in health, hair mineral analysis is a necessary part of mineral status assessment, especially used in conjunction with other tests. Foresight believes its own clinical experience belies the critics, none of whom has published credible, reliable data on this.

Hair mineral analysis and toxic metals
Hair is a reliable way to check for toxic metal levels.[22-25] (See Chapter 7.) Lead quickly passes from the blood into the bone and skeletal tissues. Cadmium rapidly disappears from the blood into other tissues, including the kidneys and liver. Hair readings correlate well with readings from these organs. Blood levels of mercury only reflect recent exposure – hair levels reflect long-term exposure. It is possible to assume no mercury toxicity from just a blood sample when, in fact, the body burden may be high.[25] With arsenic, the blood level will only increase when there is chronic toxicity, although hair and urine levels will show increases paralleling a rise in intake.[26] Aluminium hair levels are reported to be useful.[27]

Hair mineral analysis and nutrients
When it comes to the essential minerals, misunderstandings about its value arise mainly because of a lack of knowledge about interpretation.[28] If the zinc reading is high, it could mean there are high or low levels in the body. Iron levels do not seem to correlate well with body stores. But the expert recognises that since all the minerals interact with each other, it is the relationships which are reflected in the hair that must be interpreted, as well as the individual levels.[29,30] Just as a blood sample showing low iron levels could indicate a number of conditions, hair levels can do so. But no doctor would just give an iron supplement without checking that it is necessary, since the amount of iron in the diet may be quite adequate, but the patient may not have the necessary co-factors to process it. Likewise, experts will be aware of other factors when deciding on supplements of minerals with low readings on a hair analysis chart. Actually, the many practitioners around the world, including Foresight ones, who use hair mineral analysis, have shown in their clinical work that it is a reliable tool.[31-34]

Clinical observations have shown that there are typical patterns which suggest specific conditions that can then be investigated.[35,36] A useful booklet is issued by Foresight for those who need detailed information, with examples of charts.[37] The main patterns listed include the following:

○ POOR DIET PATTERN. This shows in a scatter of low minerals or low-normal minerals across the chart. The calcium may be high and zinc may be high as lack of Vitamin B6 in the diet may drive zinc into the hair causing a false high-zinc reading, while other levels may be poor.

○ ALLERGY, MALABSORPTION, REACTIVE HYPOGLYCAEMIA AND/OR CANDIDA ALBICANS. There will be low readings with some six to eight minerals below the normal range, the potassium and sodium levels being very low. This indicates adrenal stress, usually caused by a long-term allergic condition or by mental stress.[38] The reactive hypoglycaemic chart will have very high calcium, a little lower magnesium, very low sodium and potassium usually, with zinc, manganese, chromium, cobalt and/or selenium below the normal range.

People with low minerals or a ragged pattern may have a coeliac condition, cow's milk allergy or candida albicans, causing malabsorption.

○ HEAVY METAL CONTAMINATION. In this there will be high levels of one or more toxic metals. There may be adequate levels of essential elements or this may be seen with the other patterns. Minerals may be low, especially magnesium, zinc, manganese, selenium and cobalt, as the body may be using these elements to cleanse the toxins. Sodium and potassium may be high, indicating irritation of the kidneys – the levels go down after cleansing. (See Chapter 7.)

○ THE SINGLE DEFICIENCY. Where there is just one low reading, but otherwise normal levels, this will not usually indicate a dietary deficiency. The interpreter will look for an over-use of the mineral or environmental antagonists. For example:
- Low zinc may result from use of the pill or the copper IUD, from poor diet, copper contamination of drinking water, lead contamination, stress, alcohol, infection, some food additives and pesticides.
- Low magnesium may result from fluoride in drinking water.
- Low calcium often indicates an undiagnosed cow's milk allergy.
- Low manganese may indicate contamination from use of insecticides in the house, a high level of organophosphates in the food and/or use of agrochemical sprays in the locality. (See Chapter 11.)
- Low chromium and cobalt may indicate heavy consumption of sugar and/or alcohol.
- Low cobalt may be found in vegetarians and may indicate that Vitamin B12 needs supplementing.

○ DENTAL CHECK-UP. This should be done so that any treatment can be finished at least four months before conception. You should ensure that your dentist does not use amalgam fillings as these contain mercury. (See Chapter 7.) Cavities or gum infections are less likely on an adequate diet.[39]

○ DRINKING WATER SAMPLES. If your hair analysis shows high levels of copper, lead, cadmium, mercury or aluminium, you should have samples of your drinking water, both at work and home, tested to see if it contains metal contamination in excess of the World Health Organisation's allowed limits. The local Water Board has a legal obligation to test it for you if requested. If high levels are found, you should complain to the Water Board and inform the local Environmental Health Officer. You need to use a filter, and have the filtered water tested. If this also exceeds the WHO limits, you may have to consider using bottled water until the levels are restored to within the WHO limits. (Foresight recommends a Waymaster Crystal filter, with the carbon changed as advised by the manufacturer, as otherwise the carbon can become saturated, producing high levels of toxic metals.)

Conclusion

You may have thought all these tests are just too much! Your doctor may have told you that they are unnecessary. Remember, he may have qualified before the techniques were developed and he may not understand them.

BUT
- If you have had problems conceiving...
- If you have had problems with previous pregnancies...
- If you have a child who has problems...

Then you will know the anguish this can cause.

You may worry about the cost of assessment if it is not available to you on the NHS, but remember that a handicapped child is costly in both emotion and money for the whole family.

Can you afford a baby if you cannot afford the few pounds the programme costs when most of the tests are available on the NHS?

CHAPTER 5

The Vital Role of Nutrition in Pregnancy

WHAT YOU NEED TO EAT — WHY YOU NEED TO EAT IT — WHAT TO AVOID — AND HOW TO AVOID IT TO ACHIEVE A HEALTHY PREGNANCY.

If all prospective human mothers could be fed as expertly as prospective animal mothers in the laboratory, most sterility, spontaneous abortions, stillbirths, and premature births would disappear; the birth of deformed and mentally retarded babies would be largely a thing of the past.[1]

Good nutrition is the foundation of the Foresight approach to preconception care. It is vital for health, proper development and successful reproduction at all stages of life, from cells in the embryo to old age. It can help to clear the body of poisons, such as lead. It can help to protect against infection by building a healthy immune system. It is important for mental well-being.

Nutritional research

It is not always easy to do nutritional research for ethical and scientific reasons. Animal studies can provide valuable data to help understand the human situation[2] but it is not always possible to extrapolate the findings to humans. However, it has been found that in all types of animal life, from insect to mammal, a diet which supports normal adult life is insufficient to support reproduction. There is no evidence that human beings are different.[3] Examples of the similarities are apparent in the work of three pioneers in nutrition.

Three pioneers in nutrition
Some of the most remarkable research into the effects of nutrition on health was done in the 1930s by Drs Weston Price, Francis Pottenger and Sir Robert McCarrison. Although working independently, their main conclusions were the same: good health depends on good nutrition. Their research findings have never been disproved, though they have generally been ignored by the medical profession, the food industry, dieticians and governments. Those who accepted them were labelled 'cranks'. Only now is poor nutrition being recognised as a factor in ill health. NACNE[4], COMA[5], the BMA[6]

and the Health Education Council[7] have all issued recent reports which advocate changes in the national diet, though each falls short of the recommendations of our three pioneers.

Dr Weston A. Price was an American dentist who was distressed by his profession's inability to find the cause of dental caries and peridontal disease. He knew that people who did not live in civilised parts of the world had good teeth, so he travelled for ten years collecting evidence from all races of the world. His subsequent book covered many aspects of nutrition, including the vitamin and mineral content of food; soil fertility; nutrition and pregnancy; vegetarianism; the effects of processing food; and inadequate foods which produced severe degeneration. His book is not just about nutrition – it is a history of various tribes; it is an anthropological study; it is a book on agriculture, covering work that has never been written about since. Not for nothing is he known as 'The Darwin of Nutrition'.

His findings are all the more significant considering they apply regardless of the native diet he was studying. No matter who the people were, he found that as soon as they started to eat white flour and white sugar and other processed products such as tinned foodstuffs, they began to suffer ill health and there were increasing skeletal changes and other problems in the children. The actual contents of the original diets varied considerably, from the fish and seal eaten by the Eskimos, the oatmeal porridge, oatcakes and seafood of the Gaelics to the rye and milk products diet of the Loentschental Swiss. However, whatever the constituents of the original diet, when a modern diet was adopted the number of health problems increased dramatically.[8]

Dr Francis Pottenger was an American physician whose work with cats confirmed Price's findings. He observed that cats fed on scraps of raw meat were healthier than those fed on cooked meat. This led him to some remarkable research over ten years, spanning many generations and involving hundreds of cats. Basically he compared the effects of feeding one group on cooked meats, pasteurised milk and cod liver oil, and another group on raw meat, raw milk and cod liver oil. The latter group were healthy, had good skeletal structure, and reproduced healthy offspring. The former group had a high level of sickness, including allergies, birth defects, poor skeletal structure such as misshapen skull, narrow palate and jaw. They also exhibited serious behavioural problems, such as poor mothering and feeding. With each succeeding generation these problems increased. Even when placed on a raw meat diet, it took four generations of breeding before the inherited damage triggered by the cooked meat and pasteurised milk was corrected.[9]

Following these discoveries Pottenger turned to the study of human nutrition. He was particularly concerned with the effects of chemical fertilisers and processed foods, including cooked foods. He knew from his earlier work that a healthy soil was important and that this was dependent on good manure. The growth of weeds in the runs of the cats fed on raw meat, after the cats had vacated them, was luxuriant. Little growth was seen in the runs of those fed on cooked meats. Clearly, the quality of excrement, reflecting that of the diet, was an important factor in the difference. Pottenger became renowned for his work with patients, advocating the benefits of raw food in the diet.

Sir Robert McCarrison was a British doctor who served in the Indian Army, during which time he conducted many experiments in nutrition, showing how human health is dependent on the wholeness of food. Having noticed that most Sikhs, Pathans and Hunzas were healthy and well-developed, while the Bengalis and Indians in the south were disease-ridden and underdeveloped, he investigated the possible reasons using colonies of rats. Feeding them the equivalent diet of the various Indian groups, he found that each rat colony replicated the health status of the group whose diet it had been fed. He kept meticulous notes on diets, weights, health and condition at death. Those who ate a diet which deviated from the principle of eating healthy food grown on healthy soil, in as near its natural state as possible, suffered ill health. These rats had numerous diseases, reproductive failures, and behavioural problems, in one instance resorting to cannibalism. He concluded:

> I know of nothing so potent in maintaining good health in laboratory animals as perfectly constituted food; I know of nothing so potent in producing ill-health as improperly constituted food. This, too, is the experience of stockbreeders. Is man an exception to the rule so universally applicable to the higher animals?[10]

Thus, we have three men whose research findings all concluded that the quality of food was very important in good health, and for whom quality meant wholeness. If the food was treated in such a way that it lost something, by refining, tinning, or heating, health would be affected. They also all understood the importance of a healthy soil in providing good food. (See Chapter 11.)

The concept of biochemical individuality

Another important name in the history of nutrition is Dr Roger Williams, an American biochemist. In his research he found that we are all biochemically different.[11] This means that everyone has needs for levels of nutrients that are individual to them alone, especially in respect of vitamins and minerals and amino acids. It is an important principle overlooked in medical studies and dietary advice. Research has shown, for example, that some individuals may need many times the Recommended Daily Allowance (RDA) of a vitamin or mineral if they are to remain healthy.[12,13,14] In certain conditions, such as pregnancy, requirements will alter.

The importance of food before pregnancy

Although it is essential to eat properly during pregnancy, it is not enough – you need to start before conception. Good nutrition in the man helps to ensure healthy sperm and sexual activity. (See Chapter

3.) A poor nutritional status in the woman can cause problems of fertility, as birthrate studies during famines have shown.[15,16,17] (See Chapter 3.) The woman will need to have her body packed with all the nutrients the embryo will require to develop into a healthy fetus. Ideally she should be neither very overweight, nor underweight, since both can have adverse effects on pregnancy outcome.[18,19]

The importance of food during pregnancy

The work of our three pioneers has shown how important the right food is in pregnancy. Subsequent studies have confirmed this. Women on good diets have better pregnancy outcomes than those on poor diets.[20] Women who have acted upon the dietary advice they have been given also have better pregnancy outcomes than those who fail to modify their poor diets.[21] Ensuring better maternal nutrition can lower infant mortality rates.[22] The size, and maybe function, of the child's brain is dependent on good maternal nutrition.[23]

Weight gain in pregnancy

In this situation, small is NOT beautiful! Research has shown that the old idea that a woman should not put on much weight was wrong. In a London study, mothers in Hampstead who had higher calorie intakes than mothers in Hackney, had babies who were in some cases 2 lb heavier.[24] (See Chapter 3.) Dr Ebrahim, Institute of Child Health, London, found that mothers who gained more than 30 lb had the best birth outcomes.[25] Other research which has given food supplements to women has found that those who took them had bigger babies.[26] Women who are underweight at conception, and who gain less than 11 kg, or 24 lb, during pregnancy, often have babies who are small-for-date or growth retarded.

Clearly, if you eat more without exercising more you will put on weight. But it is important to eat the right foods. Besides taking in extra calories for growth and energy, you need extra vitamins, minerals, essential fatty acids, and amino acids. Moreover, if you eat the right foods, you will have less of a problem in losing the weight after birth, while breast-feeding, without a special slimming programme. You must therefore eat the most nutritious food you can. (See Chapter 11.)

A healthy diet

There are many misconceptions about a healthy diet, which have arisen mainly because we have strayed from the teachings of our three pioneers. In reviewing the importance of nutrition to preconception, Foresight originally drew from their work, and that of Roger Williams, Adelle Davis, Isobel Jennings, Eric Underwood, Lucille Hurley, Donald Caldwell and Donald Oberleas. Since then, they have continued to revise their recommendations as appropriate.

It is really quite simple to eat properly as any wholefood cookery book shows. (We recommend *The Foresight Wholefood Cookbook*,[27] which gives good basic guidance on diet and an excellent selection of recipes.)

A good diet comprises carbohydrates, fats, proteins and clean water. Within these groups are found the various vitamins and minerals that are essential for well-being. There has been so much research done on the various components that we are restricting the information in this chapter considerably, though the papers mentioned give further guidance.

○ CARBOHYDRATES should be unrefined, 'with nothing added and nothing taken away!' They include starches, sugars and fibres. They provide energy. Contrary to popular belief, they are not fattening if they are eaten in the form of complex carbohydrates. This is good news, as they are also cheap!
Good sources: Complex carbohydrates, including whole grains (wholemeal flour, millet, wholemeal bread, oatmeal, buckwheat, brown rice, maize meal), fresh vegetables and fresh fruit.
Bad sources: Simple carbohydrates, including sugars, white flour, white bread, white pasta, sweets. These are all poor in fibre, vitamins and minerals. (See Chapter 11.)

○ PROTEINS are sometimes called 'building blocks', as they are used to build or repair enzymes, muscles, organs, tissues and hair. Proteins are made of amino acids which are broken down in the body to form other amino acids. We are only just beginning to realise the potential of amino acids in health. Two amino acids, spermadine and aspermine, play a major role in the synthesis of semen.[28] Their levels have been found to be low in men who have low sperm counts. Fortunately, with the right foods and supplements, it is possible to raise the levels and help improve sperm count. Many other factors are involved in the production of healthy sperm. (See Chapters 3, 7, 8 and 10.)

Amino acids are especially important in digestion as they form the enzymes necessary for the digestive processes. Thus if they are in short supply, digestion may be affected and this may result in shortages of other nutrients in the body. Such shortages can interfere with various processes including fertility and pregnancy.[29] Animal products and fish contain all the amino acids. However, to get the full range from vegetable sources you need to combine nuts with pulses, or nuts with seeds, or pulses with seeds. Combining is an excellent way to improve the quality of protein eaten.[30,31]
Good sources: Fresh meat, poultry, offal, fish, milk, eggs, cheese, nuts, pulses and seeds (including whole grains).
Poor sources: Bought pies, TV meals, sausages and hamburgers, salamis, pâtés and other processed meats. Twice-cooked meat, as this is not fresh.

○ FATS provide energy and build the cell walls. Although animal fats are sometimes linked with illnesses such as arteriosclerosis, heart disease and some cancers, we need both animal and vegetable fats as part of a healthy diet. Eaten in the correct proportion and as part of a wholefood diet, there is no need to eliminate animal fats, such as butter, unless there is a specific medical reason. Polyunsaturated fats occur in vegetables, nuts, unheated vegetable oils and fish oils, all of which should be included in the diet. (See essential fatty acids below.) Olive oil is best for heating. You do not, therefore, generally need to eat margarines high in polyunsaturates and often highly processed! (For those who do need alternatives to butter and cream, Jervis's book is a useful source.[32])

○ WATER, if it is clean, contains useful trace elements. Sadly, much of our water does not measure up to EEC standards,[33] often having high levels of nitrates, nitrites, chemicals, lead and other toxins. (See Chapter 7.)

○ VITAMINS AND MINERALS
We make no apology for making what may seem to some readers a disproportionate coverage of vitamins and minerals. This is deliberate. The importance of these vital substances, though admitted, generally tends to be underestimated by the medical profession and dieticians. Even as long ago as 1916, a doctor wrote in the *Lancet*:
> Whatever the nature and whatever the mode of action of these puzzling substances, it is beyond question that their absence from the food does profoundly affect not only the physical health, but the mental health also.[34]

In experiments with various species, if a specific vitamin or mineral was totally omitted from the diet during the first three months of pregnancy it was found that a particular defect appeared in most of the litters, regardless of the species. Deficiencies can also affect fertility.[35,36]

Although some doctors and dieticians do not admit the necessity of vitamin and mineral supplements, there is abundant evidence on their value before and during pregnancy and during lactation.[37,38] The stores of trace elements built up by the fetus have a strong influence on the infant's copper, iron and zinc status. However, the liver does not accumulate manganese so the infant may be at risk of deficiency. The nutritional requirements of the new-born are strongly influenced by the fetal stores.[39] Such effects can be serious for the infant, since the brain continues to grow and develop very rapidly for at least two years after birth. Undernourishment, especially under four years of age, alters the brain activity and, if prolonged, can cause irreversible damage.[40] Often, it is argued that we do not know the effects of taking extra nutrients, but the many research papers in the literature disprove this. So voluminous is it that we can only concentrate below on a small proportion.

Vitamins
○ FAT-SOLUBLE VITAMINS. These include Vitamins A, D, E, K and the essential fatty acids, sometimes called Vitamin F. Because they

> **Warning**
> Foresight recommends all prospective parents and lactating mothers to supplement with the Foresight vitamins and minerals, which have been specially formulated by the Foresight medical advisers and made up by Cantassium to provide a balance of essential nutrients. Foresight does not recommend exceeding the doses suggested, or taking any megadoses, especially of individual substances, unless advised to do so by a person who is experienced in nutritional medicine, after appropriate tests.

are fat-soluble, the body can accumulate stores of them against shortages. However, in pregnancy especially, these stores may need supplementing.

Vitamin A can be obtained direct from animal products in the form of retinol, or from vegetables in the form of carotene. Carotene is then changed in the body, with the help of zinc, to proplasma Vitamin A, the form the body can use, when it is needed. If sufficient zinc is not available, it is possible to become Vitamin A deficient.[41,42]

Vitamin A is essential for healthy eyes, hair, skin, teeth, the mucous membranes, such as the lining of the mouth and good bone structure. It plays a part in good appetite, normal digestion, the making of red and white blood cells, and helps to make the hormones concerned with reproduction and lactation.

Deficiency problems in animals include increased susceptibility to infections, kidney stones, and reproductive system problems in both males and females.[43] In humans, the eyes are most affected,[44] though there are numerous reports of other conditions being helped, e.g. mental illness, skin problems, and sexual problems.[45] In the animal fetus, too little Vitamin A can result in eye defects,[46–48] hydrocephalus, diaphragmatic hernia, cleft palate and cleft lip,[49] undescended testicles,[50] and heart defects.[51] It is associated with neural tube defects in stillbirths.[52,53]

Women with diabetes mellitus have more malformed babies than women without. Problems include microcephaly, hydrocephalus, cardiac defects, and cleft palate. Vitamin A deficiency may be involved.[54]

Good sources: Vitamin A – fish oils, especially cod liver, fatty fish, egg yolk, organ meats, whole milk, butter, cream, cheese, yoghurt. Carotene – spinach, carrots, red pepper, broccoli, kale, chard, tomato, apricot, marrow, butter, cream.

It is best taken with full B–Complex, Vitamins C, D, E, essential fatty acids, calcium, phosphorus and zinc.[55]

Liquid paraffin prevents the absorption of Vitamin A, so should not be used. Long slow cooking of vegetables can destroy carotene.

Vitamin D is necessary for the growth and maintenance of bones and teeth. It also aids calcium and phosphorus absorption.[56]

Lack of Vitamin D in adults may lead to hot flushes, night sweats, leg cramps, irritability, nervousness and depression.[57,58] Other signs include osteoporosis, osteomalacia, pains in the hips and joints, and dental caries.[59] In children, rickets and tooth decay may be present. There may be other signs of bone deformities. Poor skull development can lead to impairment of brain development. Poor jaw development may give buck or snaggle teeth. It may also inhibit the function of the eustacian tubes leading to constant middle ear infection. There may be receding chins or foreheads, or large bossing foreheads with deep-set eyes. The middle face may be cramped or narrowed, pushing the palate upwards and/or forwards.[60] Price found that most retarded children and those with learning difficulties had high raised palates. Asymmetrical development of the skull may distort the membrane carrying the blood supply to the brain cells, and inlets for the blood supply may be occluded by deformed platelets. This can affect the supply of nutrients, oxygen and glucose to the brain. Girls with insufficient Vitamin D during childhood may have narrow pelvic development[61] which may make childbirth difficult.

Good sources: Vitamin D can be obtained in the food or through the action of the sun on the oils in the skin. This latter method is important, since food sources tend to be poor. Hence, it is wise to build up stores during the summer months, by allowing the action of the sun on the skin.

Food sources include fish oil and fatty fish. There are small quantities in whole milk, free range eggs and butter.

It is best taken with Vitamins A and C, choline, essential fatty acids, calcium and phosphorus.[62]

Liquid paraffin can prevent its absorption so should not be used.

Excess Vitamin D can lead to a range of unpleasant symptoms.[63]

Vitamin E prevents the oxidation (destruction by oxygen) of Vitamin A and is needed for the utilisation of essential fatty acids and selenium. It can protect from scarring after burns, surgery and injury and is important in wound healing, such as the healing of abrasions after birth.[64,65] Davies claims that some congenital heart defects will disappear if it is given from early babyhood.[66] It has also been suggested that it has a protective effect against some haemorrhage in premature babies. Researchers at the University of Edinburgh have suggested it may be another factor that can be useful in the treatment of infertility in the male, since it is necessary for flexibility in the cell walls of the sperm – abnormal sperm are less flexible.[67]

Without it people can develop anaemia, and enlarged prostate glands. Premature aging can take place with liver and kidney damage, varicose veins and heart attacks. Phlebitis, strokes, protruding eyes, muscle degeneration and muscular dystrophy can occur.[68,69]

Deficiencies in animals have caused muscular dystrophy, central nervous disorders such as encephalopathy, vascular system defects, and fetal reabsorption.[70] In rats, deficiencies lead to abnormalities including exencephaly, hydrocephalus, joined fingers and toes and oedema.[71] In human babies, they lead to anaemia, jaundice, weak muscles, retarded heart development, brain, lung and kidney damage, backward development and squint.[72]

Vitamin E may prevent miscarriage and helps to ease labour by strengthening the muscles. Prolonged labour, because of weak muscles, can lead to problems for the baby as it becomes starved of oxygen during the birth process.[73]

Good sources: Unrefined (cold pressed) oils, whole grains, wheat germ, nuts, whole milk, egg yolk, green leafy vegetables, avocado.

It is best taken with Vitamins A, full B-Complex, C, essential fatty acids, manganese, selenium.[74]

Essential fatty acids (Vitamin F) include, among others, linoleic, linolenic and arachidonic. They are important because they form a large part of the membranes of all cells, and they give rise to substances called prostaglandins. These are used to make sex and adrenal hormones and affect all systems in the body. They help in the absorption of nutrients and activate many enzymes.[75,76]

Because of the wide role of these substances in the cells, deficiencies can give rise to a large number of disorders, including allergies, gallstones, diarrhoea, varicose veins, skin problems, and heart and circulatory conditions.[77]

In reproduction, EFA deficiency may be a factor in pre-eclampsia.[78] There may be infertility, especially in the male. In rats with deficiency, the pups were of lower birth weight than was expected.[79]

Deficiencies have also been reported in hyperactive children, alcoholics and drug addicts.[80,81]

Good sources: Nuts, unrefined oils, nut butters, cold pressed, green leafy vegetables, seeds and fatty fish.

They are best taken with Vitamins A, C, D, E, and phosphorus.[82]

Vitamin K is generally made in the healthy intestine. It is essential for blood clotting, which explains why it is sometimes given to women in injection form at the time of birth. If the baby is short of this vitamin at birth, there will be a risk of bleeding, hence, it is usual to give the newly born baby an injection of it, since even small haemorrhages of the brain can be serious.[83] However, if a woman is healthy and eats plenty of green leafy vegetables, she should have a good store of the vitamin and will have a baby who has adequate stores.

○ WATER-SOLUBLE VITAMINS include the B-Complex and C. Since these are readily absorbed in water, they are easily lost to the body through urine (except B12). However, the body does have very limited stores, though any shortage is serious.

B-Complex – B vitamins should never be taken on their own, but always in conjunction with other B vitamins, because they are linked in function. Dosing with one alone may lead to a greater need for others, thereby creating a deficiency. In nature, no B vitamin is found on its own. However, it is not uncommon for a person to have a greater than usual need of any one, since we are all biochemically different.[84] (See above.)

During stress, infection, pregnancy, lactation and childhood, there is an increased need. Lack of almost any B vitamin leads to blood sugar problems in the body.

Some of the B vitamins can be made in a healthy intestine or liver, though it is not certain how much of that synthetised can be used by the body.[85,86] This does not happen where the gut is not healthy, as for example where there is a coeliac condition or candidiasis and where certain drugs (antibiotics and sulphonamides) are given. Such a condition can exacerbate any shortfall in the diet.

B-Complex is best taken with Vitamins C, E, calcium and phosphorus.[87]

Vitamin B (thiamine) is needed to break down carbohydrate into glucose.

Deficiencies lead to mental symptoms such as depression, irritability, temper tantrums, failure to concentrate and poor memory. There may be fatigue, listlessness, muscle weakness, aches and pain, anorexia, neuritis, digestion problems, heart problems and shortage of breath.[88,89]

Deficiency in animals has been linked with sterility, relative infertility,[90] low birth weight and stillbirth.[91,92] In pregnancy, it can lead indirectly to loss of appetite and vomiting, which may cause low birth weight.[93]

Good sources: Wheat germ, rice polish, whole grains, brewer's yeast, nuts, dry beans, peas, soya beans, lentils, seeds, rice, heart, kidneys.

It is best taken with full B-Complex, Vitamins C, E, manganese and sulphur.[94]

Vitamin B2 (riboflavin) assists in the breakdown and utilisation of carbohydrates, fats and proteins. It is essential for healthy eyes, mouth, skin, nails and hair. It works with enzymes in cell respiration.

Signs of deficiency are sensitivity to light, sore and bloodshot eyes, broken capillaries in the cheeks and nose, wrinkled or peeling lips and dry upper lips. There may be cracks at the corners of the mouth and dermatitis.[95,96] Experimental animals have developed cataracts, possibly because without Vitamin B2 they could not use their Vitamin A.[97] Since it works in conjunction with other nutrients and enzymes, deficiency symptoms may not disappear on straight supplementation. It should be given in conjunction with B-Complex.[98]

In animal reproduction, deficiency has been found to cause sterility, stillbirths, small misshapen fetuses, reduced oxygen consumption in the liver and reduced enzyme activity. Rats have been born with blood disorders, misshapen jaws, cleft palates, joined claws, oedema, anaemia and degeneration of the kidneys.[99] In humans, Vitamin B2 deficiency is considered to be one of the worst in pregnancy,[100] with cleft palate and shortening of limbs as risks.[101]

Good sources: Brewer's yeast, liver, kidney, tongue, leafy green vegetables, whole milk, fish, butter, cheese, peas, soya beans, legumes, blackstrap molasses, egg yolks, nuts.

It is best taken with full B-Complex and Vitamin C.[102]

Vitamin B2 is sensitive to light, so it is destroyed if milk is left on the doorstep.

Niacin or nicotinamide – sometimes known as Vitamin B3 – aids in the utilisation of energy. It is important for a healthy skin, digestive system, and the normal functioning of the gastrointestinal tract. It is also needed for proper nerve function, as a co-enzyme[103] and for the synthesis of sex hormones.[104]

Deficiencies have often been linked with the three 'D's – dermatitis, diarrhoea and dementia. There can also be a coated tongue, mouth ulcers, anorexia, dyspepsia, diarrhoea or intermittent constipation. Mental symptoms include depression, confusion, hostility, suspicion and irrational fears. Sufferers become tense, nervous, miserable, subject to dizziness, insomnia, recurring headaches and impaired memory.[105,106,107]

Nicotinamide deficiency in rats has been found to produce cleft palate and/or hare lip and hind limb defects.[108]

Good sources: Brewer's yeast, lean meats (not pork), liver, poultry, fish, brewer's yeast, wheat germ, whole grains, nuts, especially peanuts, whole milk and whole milk products.

It is best taken with full B-Complex and Vitamin C.[109]

Pantothenic acid is needed for every cell in the body as, without it, sugar and fat cannot be changed into energy. It is important for a healthy digestive tract, and essential for the synthesis of cholesterol, steroids and fatty acids and the utilisation of choline and PABA. It can help the body to withstand stress.[110]

Deficiency causes a wide variety of complaints. The adrenal glands do not function, leading to a paucity of adrenal hormones which regulate balances in the body. This may cause low blood sugar and low blood pressure. There will be a shortage of digestive enzymes, slow peristaltic action (movement along the digestive tract), indigestion and constipation following as a result. It is also linked with food allergies.[111]

As with all the B vitamins, the mental symptoms of deficiency are many, including depression, causing the sufferer to be upset, discontented and quarrelsome. There may be headaches and dizziness. These symptoms are common with low blood sugar.

In animals, deficiencies have given rise to a variety of fetal abnormalities, which mainly affect the nervous system.[112] Cleft palate, heart defects, club foot, lack of myelination, miscarriage have been noted.[113] Sterility is also mentioned.[114] Similar problems in humans are suspected.[115]

Good sources: Organ meats, brewer's yeast, egg yolks, legumes, whole grains, wheat germ, salmon, human milk, green vegetables.

It is best taken with full B-Complex, Vitamin C and sulphur.[116]

Vitamin B6 – pyridoxine – is needed to make use of the essential fatty acids and many of the amino acids. It is essential for growth and the synthesis of RNA and DNA. It helps maintain the balance of sodium and potassium in the body and is necessary for nerve and muscle function. It is needed for making nicotinamide in the liver (see above). It helps to prevent tooth decay, kidney stones, atherosclerosis and heart disease, if it is present in abundance.[117,118]

Lack of B6 can mean less use is made of minerals such as zinc, magnesium and manganese (see below). There may be headaches, halitosis, lethargy, pain and cramps in the abdomen, rash around the genitals, anaemia, anorexia, nausea, vomiting, diarrhoea, haemorrhoids, dandruff, dermatitis of the head, eyebrows and behind the ears, sore lips, tongue, and a rash round the base of the nose. Hands can become cracked and sore. Night-time problems include insomnia, twitching, tremors, leg and foot cramps and bedwetting. Mental symptoms include irritability, extreme nervousness, lethargy, and inability to concentrate.[119,120] Premenstrual tension syndrome often responds to B6 supplementation, as do nausea, vomiting, oedema and the convulsions of eclampsia in pregnancy.[121]

Fetal abnormalities, including cleft palate,[122] have been linked to B6 deficiency. Babies born with B6 deficiency have low scores on general condition ratings.[123] There may be seizures in the newborn.[124]

Good sources: meats, whole grains, organ meats, brewer's yeast, blackstrap molasses, wheat germ, legumes, peanuts.

It is best taken with full B-Complex, Vitamin C, magnesium, potassium, linoleic acid and sodium.[125]

Para-amino benzoic acid (PABA) is unique in being a 'vitamin within a vitamin', occurring in combination with folic acid.[126] It stimulates the intestinal bacteria, so they make folic acid, which is then used in the production of pantothenic acid. It helps with protein breakdown and use and in the formation of red blood cells. It is important in skin and hair colouring. It can soothe burning, especially sunburn.[127]

Good sources: brewer's yeast, wheat germ, whole grains, liver and yoghurt, organ meats, green leafy vegetables.

It is best taken with full B-Complex and Vitamin C.[128]

Biotin is necessary for the body's fat production, making fatty acids, and for the oxidation of fatty acids and carbohydrates. It also helps in the utilisation of protein, folic acid, pantothenic acid and Vitamin B12.[129] It is useful in the treatment of candidiasis.[130]

Deficiency is linked with depression, panic attacks, extreme fatigue, muscle pain, nausea, pain around the heart, dry peeling skin, hair loss, conjunctivitis, loss of appetite, pallor of skin and mucous membranes and lowered haemoglobin. In children there may be stunted growth, and adults may become thin to the point of emaciation.[131,132,133]

In rats, biotin deficiency is linked with resorption of the fetus, and death in the first few days after birth, damage to the liver, heart and blood vessels.[134]

Good sources: Egg yolks, liver, unpolished rice, brewer's yeast, whole grains, sardines, legumes.

Raw egg white destroys biotin.

It is best taken with full B-Complex, Vitamin C and linoleic acid.[135]

Inositol is needed by human liver cells and bone marrow cells. It is necessary for fat metabolism and transport, as well as healthy skin and hair. It combines with methionine and choline to make lecithin, a substance needed for the myelin sheath — the protective covering for the nerves. Lecithin also carries Vitamins A, D, E and K around the blood.

Lack of inositol may cause falling hair, eczema, abnormalities of the eyes, constipation, irregular heart action and a slowing down of the digestive system.[136,137]

Good sources: Whole grains, citrus fruits, brewer's yeast, molasses, meat, milk, nuts, vegetables and eggs.

It is best taken with full B-Complex and linoleic acid.[138]

Choline is needed for the formation of DNA and RNA and for making nucleic acid in the centre of the cell. It is used in normal muscle contraction. It is used to make lecithin (see above) and is involved in nerve functioning.

Lack of choline can lead to headaches, dizziness, strokes, haemorrhage in the eye, noises in the ear, high blood pressure, awareness of heart beat, oedema, insomnia, constipation, and visual disturbances.[139,140]

Because of its role in acetylcholine, a neurotransmitter, deficiency is linked with mental disorders, though its use in treatment is still under investigation. Animal experiments have shown a lack can cause fatty liver and haemorrhages in the heart muscle and adrenal gland.[141] It is linked with the development of stomach ulcers, liver cancer[142] and kidney damage in young animals.[143]

Insecticides, which are in common use, inactivate choline-containing enzymes, which prevents the uptake of manganese by the plants. This can then lead to manganese deficiency in the human. (See below and Chapter 11.)

Good sources: Egg yolks, organ meats, brewer's yeast, wheat germ, soya beans, fish, legumes, green vegetables.

It is best taken with Vitamins A, full B-Complex and linoleic acid.[144]

Vitamin B12 (cynocobalamin) is needed for the production and regeneration of red blood cells, and carbohydrate, protein and fat metabolism. It helps with iron function and is used with folic acid in the synthesis in choline.[145] It is involved in the synthesis of RNA and DNA.[146]

Although it is often said to occur almost exclusively in animal products, this is not true. It occurs in well water which has been exposed to the soil. Dr John Douglass also reports that, 'People who consume peanuts and sunflower seeds have adequate levels of B12. This indicates that the B12 is synthesized in the gut when the diet includes these foods. Eating seeds and sprouted seeds apparently provides the necessary nutrients to promote B12 synthesis.'[147]

Deficiency causes pernicious anaemia, deterioration of nervous tissue, sore mouth and tongue, neuritis, strong body odour, back stiffness, pain and menstrual disturbances and a type of brain damage. A very severe deficiency leads to deterioration of the spinal cord, with paralysis finally appearing.[148,149,150]

In pregnancy the fetus does not seem to be affected by variations in the mother's level. It has been noted that if several generations of rats are kept deficient, the death rate in young animals rises sharply and their weight at four weeks is reduced. The young of deficient mothers are often hydrocephalic and have eye problems.[151]

Good sources: Organ meats, fish and pork, eggs, milk, cheese, yoghurt. For vegetarians, useful quantities can be found in soy sauce, tempeh, miso, dulse, kelp, spirulina, seeds, sprouted seeds. Some types of brewer's yeast also contain small amounts.

It is best taken with full B-Complex, Vitamin C, potassium and sodium.[152]

Folic acid is needed for the formation of red blood cells in the bone marrow, the making of antibodies and the utilisation of sugars and amino acids. It is also important for the formation of nucleic acid, a substance essential for the growth and reproduction of all body cells, so it plays a crucial role in pregnancy.[153] It helps the digestive processes. It works with B12 in making haemoglobin in the blood. It is essential for zinc metabolism.[154]

Deficiency in the adult can lead to pernicious and other types of anaemia,[155] depression, dizziness, fatigue, pallor and susceptibility to infections. Anaemia in pregnancy can be a factor in smaller placentas, urinary tract infections, premature birth.[156]

Folic acid deficiency is common, and pregnancy exacerbates it. Fetal abnormalities in the young of deficient animals include cleft palate and hare lip, deformed limbs, malformations of the heart, diaphragm, urogenital system, blood vessels, adrenals, spina bifida, malformations of the eye, skeletal deformities, underdevelopment of the lung and kidney, cataracts, brain deformities, oedema, and anaemia.[157] Fetal death and miscarriage or resorption may occur.[158] If folic acid is given at the time of resorption, the fetus may survive to term but may have hydrocephalus.[159]

If deficiency occurs during pregnancy, microcephaly can be seen in the new born rats.[160]

In humans, folic acid has been the subject of much attention in pregnancy, especially in relation to neural tube defects, such as spina bifida. A number of studies have been done which suggest that women who are given supplements of folic acid in the month before conception and for the first 8–10 weeks afterwards, are less likely to have a malformed baby.[161,162,163] Many of the research methods used in the studies have been criticised as not proving the value of folic acid supplements, and in some cases the points made are valid. But it is unethical to do the sort of study that the critics want, because it would mean giving one group of women folic acid and a second group a placebo tablet without folic acid and seeing if the latter group had more deformed babies. Some people argue that this is not necessary – the differences between incidence of neural tube defects in the control population and the women taking the tablets is so marked that there could not be any other likely explanation, other than that the supplement had made the difference.[164] The double-blind experiment which met the criticisms of the earlier studies did not show significant differences between those women taking the supplement and those on the placebo. But two women in the supplemented group who had babies with a neural tube defect probably did not take their tablets.[165] The Medical Research Council has started another trial which is scientifically correct in its design but which has met much criticism. Many medical centres have refused to participate since they believe that it would be unethical not to give women the vitamin supplement in view of the evidence from other studies. The supplement used was Pregnavite Forte F, which is formulated as a dose of one a day. Taking three in a day, as happened in some of the experiments, brings the total Vitamin A content to 12,000 i.u., which is more than is recommended.

A further study has suggested that supplements before pregnancy would be protective.[166]

Taking the research into account, there seems little doubt that folic acid deficiency in the mother, especially in the early stages of pregnancy, can be a major contributory factor in neural tube defects. Many other types of malformations were seen in animal studies.

Good sources: Green leafy vegetables, brewer's yeast, organ meats, whole grains, wheat germ, milk, salmon, root vegetables, nuts.

It is best taken with full B-Complex and linoleic acid.[167]

Vitamin C keeps the collagen (connective tissue) healthy and resistant to penetration by viruses, poisons, toxins such as lead, dangerous drugs, allergens, and/or foreign materials. It promotes healing after surgery, infection or injury, including broken bones. It keeps the capillary walls intact. It helps the absorption of iron, preventing anaemia. It is important for mental health.[168,169,170]

Deficiency symptoms include scurvy, dandruff, haemorrhages on the thighs, buttocks and abdomen, swollen and bleeding gums, leading to infection, ulceration and lose of teeth. There may be spontaneous bleeding. Children who are short of Vitamin C are prone to infections, have poor teeth and gums. Their bones break easily, they bruise easily and quickly tire and become irritable.[171] It has been linked with miscarriage.[172]

Good sources: Citrus fruits, rose hips, sprouted alfalfa seeds, tomatoes, green peppers, broccoli and other green vegetables, blackcurrants, strawberries and other soft fruits, bananas, apples, pears, carrot, cauliflower, new potatoes eaten with their skins – Vitamin C is lost in storage, parsley.

It is best taken with all vitamins and minerals, bioflavenoids, calcium and magnesium.[173]

Minerals
Calcium is needed for the formation of strong bones and teeth, and for controlling blood clotting mechanisms and proper nerve and muscle function. Other functions include assisting in muscle growth, maintaining blood balance and acting as a catalyst in enzyme reactions.[174,175,176] It may help to protect against allergies, viruses and tooth decay.[177]

In pregnancy, calcium is vital for the growth of the fetus and the well-being of the mother. Davis recommends giving it, in conjunction with Vitamin D, during labour to ease pain.[178] It can ease leg cramps.[179,180] Low levels are associated with low birth weight and low scores on developmental tests.[181] Premature babies tend to have low levels.[182] Calcium is lost from the bones during bedrest and also while on high protein diets. People affected will need to supplement the diet and to choose foods with high levels.

Lack of calcium can cause rickets, back pain, osteoporosis, osteomalacia, irritability, nervousness, tension, uneven heartbeat, indigestion, stomach cramps and spasms, constipation, premenstrual tension, and cramping of the uterus.[183,184]

Good sources: Kelp, cheese, carob, bone broth, green vegetables, brazil nuts, whole raw milk (pasteurisation reduces calcium availability), dolomite, brewer's yeast, yoghurt.

Foods containing oxalic acid (sesame seed hulls, rhubarb, spinach) and phytic acid (soda and unleavened bread) can reduce availability.

It is best taken with Vitamins A, C, D, essential fatty acids, iron, magnesium, phosphorus.[185]

Chromium is needed for the regulation of the glucose tolerance factor, in combination with nicotinic acid and some proteins. Glucose is required for every bodily function – it is the body's fuel. Chromium is also necessary for the synthesis of fatty acids and cholesterol. A deficiency may be linked with heart disease.[186]

Chromium is not easily absorbed, though it is readily removed from the body. Even a small deficiency will be serious.

Good sources: Brewer's yeast, black pepper, liver, whole grains, wheat germ, vegetables, butter, beer, molasses.

Cobalt is an essential part of Vitamin B12 (see above). There is a possible relationship between cobalt and iodine.[187] It is necessary in B12 for the normal functioning of all cells, but especially red blood cells, and has been used in the treatment of pernicious anaemia. However, there are serious toxic side effects so its role is of limited value.[188] It activates some enzymes.[189] Deficiency is associated with pernicious anaemia[190] and maybe with slow growth[191] and goitre.[192]

Good sources: Although it is said that cobalt can only be taken by humans in the form of Vitamin B12, Underwood points out that organ meats and muscle meats each contain more than can be accounted for as Vitamin B12.[193] Green leafy vegetables are a rich source if the soil was rich, but others include meats, brewer's yeast, seafoods, nuts, fruit and whole grains.

Cobalt is more effective when taken with copper, iron and zinc.[194]
Copper aids the development of brain, bones, nerves and connective tissue. It is involved in many enzyme systems, and is essential in the production of RNA.[195,196]

Deficiency can cause porous bones, loss of hair, demyelination, heart damage and anaemia.[197]

In the fetus of a number of animals, copper deficiency can result in depressed growth rate, depigmentation, anaemia, fine, fragile bones, ataxia, small brain and perinatal mortality. In rats, infertility has been noted.[198] Skeletal and cardiovascular defects, central nervous system disorders, and steely wool hair (failure of melanin formation) have also been reported.[199]

Copper deficiency is rare, and copper in excess can be toxic. (See Chapter 7.)

Good sources: Shellfish, brazil nuts, organ meats, dried legumes, dried stone fruits and green vegetables.

It is best taken with cobalt, iron and zinc.[200]

Iodine is necessary for the formation of thyroxine and triiodothyronine, hormones produced by the thyroid. Thyroxine is necessary for growth, mental and physical development and the maintenance of health. Most people are aware that too little iodine can cause goitres, but deficiency is also associated with fatigue, lethargy, susceptibility to cold, loss of interest in sex,[201] slow development of the sex organs, anorexia, slow pulse, low blood pressure, rapid weight gain, high blood cholesterol,[202] death from heart disease and cancer of the thyroid.[203]

Deficiency in the pregnancy can result in cretinism in children, a congenital disease with mental and physical retardation.[204] If iodine is given soon after birth, many of the symptoms are reversible.[205]

Good sources include water, iodised salt, watercress, onions, kelp, shellfish, and mushrooms and dark leafy vegetables if they are grown on soil rich in iodine.

Too much iodine can also have serious consequences for health.[206]

Iron is needed to make haemoglobin, the substance in the red blood cells, which carries oxygen in the blood. It also aids resistance to infection. It helps supply oxygen to the muscles. It helps in protein digestion and also in respiratory function.[207]

Needs in pregnancy increase because the number of red blood cells increases by 30 per cent. Since most women do not have a large enough store before pregnancy, the small amounts of iron in the diet may not be sufficient, so many women are given supplements. This can be quite unsatisfactory if other nutrients are not given, since iron is not absorbed well without Vitamin C and needs to work with other vitamins and minerals.[208,209] Iron given alone can also cause loss of other essential minerals, such as zinc, manganese, chromium, selenium and cobalt.

Shortage of iron can lead to weakness, excessive fatigue, depression, headache, pallor, lack of appetite, mental confusion and poor memory.[210–213] Iron-deficient people will absorb two to three times more lead than non-deficient people.[214] (See Chapter 7.) Deficiency is not so common in men, but it does occur in children, particularly if they are eating a diet which includes white flour and white sugar.

In the fetus, iron deficiency can cause eye defects, slow growth, bone defects, brain defects and neonatal mortality.[215]

Good sources: Organ meats, liver, kelp, brewer's yeast, molasses, wheat germ, almonds, parsley, egg yolk, lean meats, whole grains, vegetables.

The iron of egg yolk is poorly absorbed unless taken with a food containing Vitamin C. Thus, a glass of fresh orange juice with an egg is a good source of iron.

Blood donors of both sexes are at risk of iron deficiency, so giving blood when you are planning a pregnancy should be avoided.

The usual test for iron is using blood. However, since the body will draw on its stores from the tissues and bone to maintain the amount circulating in the body, blood is not the best way of checking levels. For this reason, some doctors prefer to use hair samples as well.

Magnesium is needed for the production and transfer of energy, muscle contraction, proper nerve function, protein synthesis and the functioning of many enzymes.[216]

Deficiencies cause involuntary muscle movements, such as spasms and twitching, convulsions, insomnia, irregular heartbeat, leg and foot cramps, bedwetting and depression.[217,218] Pregnancy aggravates any deficiency.

A deficiency is said to contribute to painful uterine contractions at the end of pregnancy. It may also be associated with miscarriage or premature birth.[219] Rats fed low magnesium diets give birth to smaller pups with a higher rate of congenital deformities. They also develop calcium deposits and other abnormalities in the heart cells.[220] Women with low levels tend to abort more or have low birth weight babies.[221,222]

Good sources: Nuts, kelp, green vegetables, seafoods, eggs, milk, whole grains, dolomite.

Magnesium is best taken with Vitamins B6, C, D, calcium, phosphorus, protein.[223]

Manganese is needed for numerous enzyme reactions, bone growth and development, lipid metabolism, and nerve function. It is necessary in the formation of thyroxine (see iodine) and in blood clotting.[224,225] It may contribute to a mother's maternal instincts and love, through its role in certain enzymes.[226]

Although its function in reproduction is not understood, there is no doubt that a deficiency can affect fetal development. In rats it has been shown that in the least severe stage there is an increase in the number of offspring born with ataxia. In the second, more serious stage, the young are born dead or die shortly after birth, while in the third, most serious stage, the animal will not mate, and sterility results. This is also seen in hens.[227] In the male rat and rabbit with severe deficiency there is sterility, and also absence of sex drive, associated with degeneration of the seminal tubes and lack of spermatozoa.[228,229] In the young there may be faulty cartilage and bone matrix formation and heart and neural function problems.[230] Animals from mothers who are deficient show difficulty with behavioural tasks.[231]

Good sources: Nuts, whole grains, seeds, leafy green vegetables, brewer's yeast, egg, liver, parsley, thyme, cloves, ginger, tea (but see Chapter 8).

It is best taken with Vitamins B1, E, calcium, phosphorus.[232]

Uptake of manganese is inhibited by choline deficiency. (See choline above.)

Nickel is found in high concentrations in DNA and RNA and in all tissues and fluids. Most of the work on it has been focused on animals. It is needed for the action in the enzyme urease.[233] In studies, deficiencies have been linked with reproductive failures and growth problems.[234] In the rat, it is associated with the metabolism of copper and manganese. It may have a role in hormonal control[235] and as an enzyme co-factor.[236] High levels are found in the blood of patients who have suffered heart attacks.[237] It is thought that the damaged heart muscles release the nickel. Low levels are decreased in those with cirrhosis of the liver, or chronic uremia.[238] Deficiency is claimed to have a negative influence on growth and life expectancy[239] and to impair iron metabolism.[240]

Good sources include soya beans, dry beans, lentils, nuts, buckwheat, grains and vegetables.

Sources not recommended: It is also found in hydrogenated vegetable oils, such as corn, as it is used as a catalyst in the processing.[241]

Too much nickel can also have serious health risks.[242]

Phosphorus is the second most abundant mineral in the body, being found in every cell. As it functions with calcium, both being the main constituents of bone, it is important that its balance with calcium is maintained. It plays a part in almost every chemical reaction in the body, in the utilisation of carbohydrates, proteins and fats, in muscle and nerve function, digestion, kidney function, and proper skeletal growth. It is found in important substances called phospholipids, which break up and transport fats and fatty acids. (See essential fatty acids above.) Among their many functions are the promotion of the secretion of glandular hormones.[243,244]

Deficiency is rare, since it is found in artificial fertilisers.[245] (See Chapter 11.) It is also a common ingredient in many food additives (yet another reason for avoiding them!) and soft drinks. The right way to ensure balancing it with calcium and other minerals is to obtain it from the whole foods.

Good sources: Brewer's yeast, whole grains, bread, cereals, meat, fish, poultry, eggs, seeds, nuts.

Phosphorus is best taken with Vitamins A, D, essential fatty acids, calcium, iron, manganese, protein.[246]

Potassium is needed to regulate blood pH, to acidify urine, and for proper nerve and muscle functioning. It is involved in the utilisation of enzymes. It may be involved in bone calcification. Together with sodium, it maintains the fluid balance in the body and may help in the transportation of nutrients into the cells.[247] It is necessary for growth.[248]

A deficiency causes nervous irritability, insomnia, oedema, headaches, irregular heart beat, bone and joint pain, constipation, cramping of muscles, weakness and fatigue. In the embryo, it may cause abnormalities in the kidneys.[249] Deficiency may result from too much sodium chloride (salt), too little fruit and vegetables, some diseases and some medical treatments.[250]

Potassium chloride has been used successfully in the treatment of children's colic and diarrhoea in adults as well as children.[251]

Good sources: Brewer's yeast, wheat germ, whole grains, vegetables, fruit, nuts.

Potassium is best taken with Vitamin B6, sodium.[252]

Selenium, like Vitamin E with which it is associated in some functions, is a powerful anti-oxidant which helps to prevent chromosomal damage in tissue culture. Such damage is associated with birth defects and cancers. It is a vital part of an important enzyme which helps the body to fight infections. In animals and chickens, deficiencies are associated with slow growth, cataracts, infertility, loss of hair and feathers, degeneration, nutritional muscular dystrophy, swelling and haemorrhages, pancreatic atrophy, and liver necrosis.[253,254] In human cell culture it is required for growth, so it may be necessary for normal growth. Selenium will combine with toxic metals, such as cadmium, so it is useful for detoxifying. It may be important in preventing cot deaths. In the USA about a quarter of the babies who die each year are found to be deficient in selenium and/or Vitamin E. Most of them were bottle-fed.[255]

Good sources: Butter, smoked herring, wheat germ, brazil nuts, brewer's yeast, whole grains, garlic and liver. For the baby, human milk is an excellent source.

Selenium can also be toxic, though. Foresight practitioners have found excesses in people who use selenium-containing anti-dandruff shampoos in the bath, and then soak in the water. It is possible that some Xerox copying machines can also produce selenium in the atmosphere.

Selenium is more effective when taken with Vitamin E.[256]

Silicon is critical in the formation of connective tissues, bones, the placenta, arteries and skin, keeping it impermeable. It has been found to be essential for growth and skeletal development in rats and chicks.[257,258]

Good sources: Whole grains, wholemeal bread, alfalfa, vegetables, especially the skins, pectin and hard water.

Vanadium is present in most tissues in the body and is rapidly excreted into urine. It is thought to exert some influence on lipid metabolism by inhibiting cholesterol formation.[259] It is part of the natural circulatory regulating system. Raised levels are possibly involved in the aetiology of manic depressive psychosis.[260] Deficiency in animals results in impaired bone development, reduced growth, and disturbance of blood metabolism, decreased reproduction and increased perinatal mortality, and reduced fertility in subsequent generations.[261,262]

Good sources: buckwheat, parsley, soya beans, eggs, sunflower seed oil, oats, olive oil, olives, rice, green beans, vegetables.

Zinc is needed for the health and maintenance of hormone levels, bones, muscles and sperm. It is important in healing. It is needed for the functioning of at least 200 enzymes.[263] It is an important component of semen.[264] It is necessary to stabilise RNA.[265] It is needed in Vitamin A metabolism. (See Vitamin A above.) It is essential for brain development and function.[266,267] Caldwell and Oberleas have shown in rats that 'even a mild zinc deficiency has a potential influence on behaviour potential despite an apparently adequate protein level in the diet'.[268]

In the male, zinc can increase the size of the penis and testes in growing boys. It also increases sperm motility[269] (see Chapter 3) and helps to prevent impotence.[270]

Lack of zinc is associated with a loss of the senses of taste and smell, both of which affect appetite and anorexia.[271] In animals, eye problems, high rates of miscarriage (resorption), brain malformation, cleft palate, cleft lip, club feet, stillbirth and urinary-genital abnormalities have been found.[272] Low levels in maternal rats have been associated with learning problems[273] and behavioural problems[274] in their offspring. With all the concern about a general weakening of the immune system, it is worrying to note that in an experiment with mice, damage occurred to the immune system of offspring whose mothers were zinc deficient. The damage persisted even when supplements of zinc were given.[275]

Low zinc status in the mother is a factor in infertility,[276] and low birth weight.[277] Low plasma levels at mid-pregnancy have been associated with more complications at delivery[278] and a higher incidence of malformations.[279] Deficiency also inhibits Vitamin A metabolism. (See Vitamin A above.) Children suffer more allergies and more infections.[280] Deficiencies have been found in children with learning disabilities, especially dyslexia.[281] Low levels were found in the hair of children suffering from anorexia, poor growth and hypogeusia (loss of taste).[282]

Good sources: Oysters, whole grains, meat, brewer's yeast, wheat germ, fruit, vegetables, nuts, offal, fish, poultry, shellfish. It is best taken with Vitamin A, calcium, copper and phosphorus.[283]

Food purchase and preparation

Knowing the contents of a healthy diet, you want to ensure that you do not spoil them by the wrong sort of preparation. Again, a good wholefood cookery book will help but there are some very basic guidelines. (See Chapter 11.)

- Buy organically grown produce where possible.
- Buy fresh before frozen.
- Eat as much food as you can in its raw state – most vegetables and fruit are delicious raw.
- Steam rather than boil.
- Stir fry rather than deep fry.
- Grill, roast or stew rather than fry.
- Prepare food as near to eating as possible.

Conclusion
It is often said that 'We are what we eat', and, like most clichés, there is an element of truth in it. If we want to be healthy, we must eat healthy food. If we want to have healthy children, we must recognise that this means providing the best ingredients – that is, the best food. This means food which is grown on good soil, or reared in healthy conditions, and eaten as near its natural state as possible. Fortunately, there is an increasing awareness that organic produce is superior and it is becoming more available. Enjoy it, knowing that this was the type of food our three pioneers found to promote well-being and productive success! But also recognise that with modern life-styles, it is unlikely to give you all you need to prepare for pregnancy and lactation – you will need to supplement it.

CHAPTER 6

Planning Your Family the Natural Way

THE METHOD THAT SAFEGUARDS YOUR HEALTH AND FUTURE FERTILITY, WHILE YOU PLAN YOUR FAMILY.

The Foresight way to have a baby means *planning* the right time to conceive, when both partners are healthy, so you will need to give careful consideration to birth control. There are a number of methods available and the choice can seem bewildering until the facts about each are reviewed. It then becomes apparent that there are methods which are not health-promoting, especially for the woman, since they can have serious side effects. (See Chapter 9.) In this chapter, we explain how you can plan your family safely, using natural family planning (NFP) and/or barrier methods. Foresight recommends natural family planning, with either abstention or the use of a barrier method on fertile days, although recognising that some couples may prefer to use barrier methods all the time. However, except in a few cases, this is unnecessary, as there are only a few days in each monthly cycle when a woman is fertile. Moreover, a main advantage of NFP used on its own is that it teaches fertility awareness and this can be important when a couple have fertility problems.

Natural family planning

Pregnancy can only occur when an active sperm meets an egg that is ready to be fertilised. Since the egg can only survive for up to 24 hours and the sperm can survive for three to six days, it follows that pregnancy can only happen if intercourse takes place during the vulnerable seven days in each monthly cycle. Natural family planning methods aim to identify these days so that a couple can either take measures to avoid pregnancy or use the knowledge to conceive. Throughout history people have linked times in the cycle with fertility – not always the right time! Misunderstandings have led to loss of confidence in various methods, especially the rhythm method (calendar method), widely recommended in the past for Roman Catholics. NFP is *not* a rhythm method and should never be confused with it, although you will find many, including doctors, who do equate the two methods. Modern NFP is derived from the latest knowledge about the monthly cycle, the same on which the contraceptive pill was developed – but there the similarity ends.

The advantages of NFP have been listed by Dr Anna Flynn, a leading expert. They include: no known side effects; more awareness of fertility, which helps promote a more responsible attitude to family planning and sometimes a better relationship between partners; a morally acceptable and viable method for those for whom abstinence but not other methods are suitable; and personal control over fertility. Once taught, there is no need for follow-up or further expenses; it can help achieve pregnancy.[1]

Like every other method there are disadvantages, including a failure rate which may be as low as one per cent or up to 20–30 per cent depending on which study is quoted. Flynn identifies three important factors which contribute to success or failure:

1. *Motivation.* More success is reported among users who want to limit their families than among those who are spacing pregnancies or delaying them.
2. *Efficient teaching.* Success depends on identifying the fertile period and this is best taught by competent teachers, ideally to both partners.
3. *Characteristics of the woman.* Some find it difficult to identify the various types of mucus, though one researcher found that 97 per cent could do so correctly.[2] Others do not like touching themselves. If abstinence is the option, it may be hard at a time when, for many, libido is high.

We firmly believe that NFP needs to be taught properly and for that reason we shall not be giving a 'do-it-yourself guide'. In Appendix One we do give addresses where you can find a teacher. What we do below is explain the theory behind the method.

Basically there are three main ways of identifying the fertile days:
1. Checking the mucus.
2. Checking the cervix.
3. The temperature method.

In practice, you will be advised to use at least 1 and 2 together or, preferably, all three to obtain maximum reliability.

Checking the mucus

This method (and checking the cervix) can tell you when the egg is about to be released (ovulation). It is important to be able to calculate in advance when this will take place since sperm can survive in the vagina for three or even five days around the time of ovulation. At other times they die within a few hours as they cannot live in the usually acidic environment of the vagina. Early in the cycle, several eggs begin to ripen in the ovary, producing increasing amounts of oestrogen, the female sex hormone. Oestrogen causes the production of mucus from the cervix, mucus which helps the sperm to survive in the vagina, and to travel to meet the egg when it is released at ovulation. After menstruation, the vagina and vulva feel dry, because little mucus is being released. The level of oestrogen is low, and the mucus is cloudy, thick, sticky and so is able to stop the sperm from entering the womb. However, as the level of oestrogen rises, it becomes more watery, clear and, like egg-white, slippery and stretchy. The vagina and vulva feel moist or wet, and the vagina becomes alkaline, just as the sperm like it. Sometimes mid-cycle bleeding occurs and the mucus is pinkish. The last day of fertile mucus is called 'Peak Day', as it is the day when ovulation is most likely to occur. After ovulation the mucus dries up again to form a plug in the cervix which stops any sperms getting through in case there has been a fertilisation. The first three days after Peak Day are regarded as fertile days, to allow for the release, life and death of the egg and the complete reforming of the mucus plug. The rest of the cycle is infertile. It is easy to observe the mucus when you visit the toilet by wiping the vulva with toilet paper. You should also observe your subjective feelings of wetness or dryness, ideally noting them on the chart on which you record your temperature. (See below.)

Checking the cervix

Not only does the mucus change throughout the cycle, so does the state of the cervix, the changes correlating with those in the mucus. It is all very logical. At the time when the egg is ready to be fertilised, the mouth of the cervix opens to help the sperm meet the egg. When the egg is not ready to be fertilised, it closes to stop the sperm from entering the womb. You can feel these changes, though sometimes if you have already had a baby the cervix never does fully close.

The cervix is at the upper end of the vagina – a cylindrical shape about an inch in diameter. The best time to learn to check it is late in the infertile phase when it is at its lowest point in the vagina. At this time, it will be firm, with the mouth closed. The surface will be dry and may be gritty. As you move towards fertility, it changes, softening like ripening fruit. It gets soft and sticky as the mucus forms. In the fertile phase it is higher up in the vagina, soft, rubbery, slippery, and the mouth, or os, is fully open. After the fertile phase, it reverts to its low, firm, closed state.

The temperature method

This depends on the rise and fall in temperature that occurs throughout the cycle, as the body warms up to act as a natural incubator if fertilisation occurs. When the egg is released the woman's temperature may drop very slightly, which is noticeable using a special fertility thermometer. Immediately afterwards, because of the release of progesterone (another hormone) the temperature of the body at complete rest rises between 0.2–0.4°C, staying at the new higher level until the start of the next period. When it has been at the higher level for three days, it is unlikely that the egg will be fertilised by any sperm which may still be present.

To use this method the woman must take her temperature on waking up, before getting up, or having a drink, using a fertility thermometer. The result is recorded on a fertility chart. (See Appendix One for useful addresses from which to obtain thermometers and charts.) She must also record any factor that could have disturbed her temperature, as taught by her NFP teacher. Such factors could include lack of sleep, shock, travel or shift work to mention but a few. Drugs such as aspirin can lower body temperature, confusing the chart. A high temperature for more than 20 days may mean a pregnancy – indeed, it is the earliest objective indicator.

The disadvantage of the method is that it cannot tell when ovulation is going to occur and when the fertile phase starts. This is why it should be used in conjunction with the mucus method. An NFP teacher will show how the methods complement each other to provide a highly reliable and safe method of family planning.

Aid in natural family planning
There are a number of aids that can be bought to help detect the infertile period. Most test the level of Luteinising Hormone in the urine. It is this hormone which triggers ovulation. For those who have entered the computer age, there is OVIA, which the inventor claims is the first electronic fertility assessor. We have not tested it, though the theory, as explained in a book by the inventor, seems sound.[3] (See Appendix One for addresses.)

Barrier methods
Condom (Also known as sheath, protective, rubber, French letter.) Having fallen from popularity with the advent of the pill and IUD, the condom is now very much in favour, because it is the only method of contraception which is recommended as offering some protection against sexually transmitted diseases (including AIDS) and possibly cancer of the cervix. Used *properly* it is a highly effective contraceptive, up to 98 per cent reliable, especially if combined with a spermicide (see below). The usual reason for failure is improper use, particularly in putting it on, or not being careful in holding it on withdrawing from the vagina. Easily obtained, and free from family planning clinics, it is also the only method for which the man is responsible. It does not need medical advice and there are very few complications. Thus most people can use it, although some may not like the interruption of love-making that may result, unless its use is incorporated in love-play. Some pleasurable sensation may be lost.

Diaphragm (Also known as the cap.)
There are a number of caps, the most common being the diaphragm. Others include the cervical and vault caps which are held over the cervix by suction – the diaphragm is held by spring tension. They may be fitted where the diaphragm is unsuitable. All work by preventing the sperm from reaching the cervix, but since women's shapes vary so much and alter during intercourse you should always use a spermicide. You will need to be measured for a diaphragm and shown how to use it. For the highly motivated couple it can be very

reliable – up to 97 per cent. Failure is normally associated with incorrect insertion or fitting, or defects through improper handling. It may protect against cancer of the cervix.[4] Since it can be inserted at any convenient time before intercourse, spontaneity is possible, although this means some planning is necessary. There may be a loss of cervical and some vaginal sensation.

Honeycap
This is a special diaphragm, impregnated with honey, a natural anti-microbe agent. It can thus be left in the vagina overnight. It is said not to need spermicides. However, little information is available on it, including reliability figures, so we cannot recommend it.

Sponge
This is a foam sponge impregnated with spermicide which can be inserted in the vagina up to 24 hours before intercourse. It must be left in for six hours afterwards to ensure that all the sperm are killed. It does not need special fitting and intercourse can be repeated within the 24 hour period, after which it is thrown away – it can, therefore, be expensive compared with other methods. It works in the same way as the diaphragm, by stopping the sperm from reaching the egg. Reliability, with careful use, is claimed to be up to 90 per cent. However, one study found a failure rate up to 24.5 per cent.[5]

Spermicide
Spermicides work by the use of a base material which physically blocks the progression of sperm, and a chemical which is designed to kill the sperm without damaging other body tissues. However, in some cases, they can irritate one or both partners. They come in five main forms:

1. Creams and jellies.
2. Vaginal pessaries which spread less easily throughout the vagina so are probably less effective than creams and jellies.
3. Foaming tablets.
4. Aerosol foams, which should not be used with the cap.
5. C-film – a square of water-soluble plastic, impregnated with spermicide, which is placed high in the vagina.

Spermicides should not be used on their own. They are best regarded as a back-up to other barrier methods. We would suggest that creams, jellies and foaming tablets are the preferred spermicides.

○ IN SUMMARY. If it is taught by a trained teacher and properly done, NFP is as effective as the pill in preventing pregnancy. It is also the only method that can be used to plan the most likely days to become pregnant.

When deciding which, if any, barrier method to use during the fertile days, you should remember that they are all much more effective when used with care, but they are still not 100 per cent reliable at the most fertile time. Only abstention is absolutely safe!

PART FOUR

Negative influences on preconception and prenatal health

CHAPTER 7

Problems in the Twentieth Century: Toxic Metals

INFORMATION TO HELP YOU SAFEGUARD YOUR BABY BY AVOIDING TOXINS — AND WHY YOU NEED TO DO SO.

All trace elements can be toxic if consumed in sufficient quantities. However, the term 'toxic metals' generally denotes 'those elements not recognised as having an essential function and known to have well documented deleterious effects'.[1] It is these on which we focus in this chapter.

Although man has been utilising many of them for hundreds of years, in this century their use has escalated as new processes, purposes and products have been developed. As a result, we now have more widespread pollution than ever before, with concomitant problems. Even though we know there are adverse effects of lead ingestion and inhalation, we are still reluctant to change to unleaded petrol. We are aware of the dangers of cadmium, highlighted in discussions on high soil levels, yet we overlook the major sources, cigarette smoking and refined flours. Dentists have been aware of the dangers of mercury for many years, but still use mercury containing amalgams. We are now being told that aluminium may be a factor in Alzheimer's Disease – yet we know that patients in mental hospitals imbibe large amounts of tea which contains high levels of aluminium! It would seem prudent to assume that aluminium is toxic, until we know otherwise. At the least, this would not harm anyone, and at the best, it could save many from hospitalisation, if it is true. A major shift needs to take place from the assumption that a substance is safe until it is proven otherwise, to the position that it is dangerous until proved safe!

There is also a dearth of studies which look at more than one element, even though it is known that there is continual interaction between many of them. Fortunately, the work of Bryce-Smith and Ward, among others, is remedying this, though such research is difficult and expensive.[2]

In this chapter, we examine the data on lead, cadmium, mercury, aluminium, copper and some other elements on which there has been less research. Since all chemicals interact in the body, we pay special attention to the studies which cover more than one metal, especially lead and cadmium, before explaining how the body can be detoxified.

Lead

The single most researched chemical, lead has been known to be toxic to animals and humans for centuries. Despite this, its use has increased dramatically, especially in the last 40 years, so that it is now impossible to escape ingesting or inhaling it. It comes mainly from the atmosphere, polluted by exhaust fumes from lead in petrol and from food, especially that grown in soils polluted by lead from petrol, and unlined cans.[3,4] A London GP warned against eating food grown in London.[5] Water which has coursed through old lead piping, or through lead-glazed earthenware mains, or through modern copper piping where the joins of the pipes have been formed with lead-containing alloys, is also a major source for many people. Cigarette smoking can increase lead uptake by 25 per cent, partly because of the way it interacts with other substances, and also from the lead arsenate used as an insecticide for tobacco.[6,7] Occupational exposure can be a hazard, as lead is used in a number of industries.[8,9] High rates of infertility, miscarriage, stillbirth, congenital abnormalities including macrocephaly, convulsions, early deaths and chromosomal alterations have been reported.[10,11] Children are at greater risk than adults, because they ingest more and have immature bodies. But lead can also cross the placenta, and so affect the fetus. The younger the child, the greater the risk, since lead affects the brain and the greatest brain development occurs before and in the first few years after birth.[12]

Animal research suggests that nutritional status may be a factor in lead absorption. Diets low in calcium, iron, zinc and manganese may actually enhance lead uptake. However, one study also suggests that cow's milk may increase absorption, since, although high in calcium, it is low in other trace minerals such as iron.[13] The fact that lead can be removed from the body by nutrients further supports the idea that nutritional status is important. (See below.)

There is, as yet, no agreement on safety levels. Some researchers say that no level can be assumed to be safe, while the government sets limits for industry and the environment which are lowered from time to time as more is revealed about its toxicity.[14] There are no agreed ways to measure levels, which adds to the problem. Blood lead levels are not reliable, as the lead is passed from the blood to other tissues, especially bones, quite quickly. Hair analysis, though accepted as a reliable guide, is not widely available. (See Chapter 4.)

But, regardless of the arguments, there is no longer any doubt that levels which do not manifest symptoms of 'classical' poisoning may have subtle effects on the body. Chronic 'low' level lead exposure is implicated as a significant causative or contributory factor in a wide range of conditions, including cardiovascular disease, renal and metabolic disease, immune dysfunction, and a multiplicity of vague symptoms, such as lethargy, depression, muscle aches and pains, frequent infections, cancer, developmental abnormalities and learning, behavioural and central nervous system dysfunction.[15,16] Lead interferes with the normal functioning of many trace elements, especially by inhibiting zinc dependent enzymes, making its effects widespread.[17] Other enzyme systems are also vulnerable. High childhood blood levels and smaller stature have been shown to be highly correlated.[18]

Lead and the next generation
Lead can affect both male and female reproductive abilities. Men exposed to high levels in their work have been found to be at risk of low sperm count, with more sperm likely to be misshapen and less mobile.[19,20] In women, its capacity for inducing abortions has long been known – it was used around the turn of the century with, sometimes, blindness and brain damage in surviving babies. It was also this property that ensured women were not being employed to work with lead.[21] One reason it may be abortifacient lies in its tendency to accumulate in the placenta.[22]

Research in the 70s has linked high lead levels with stillbirth. In 1977, a study of placental lead levels showed that there were greater amounts in the placentas of malformed stillbirths and neonatal deaths compared with normal births surviving longer than a week.[23] In the same year, two other researchers reported higher levels of lead (and cadmium – see below) in stillbirths, using rib and pre-ossified cartilage for the analyses. They concluded: 'Although some levels were low, others were so high as to raise the suspicion that they were aetiologically connected with the death of the fetus.'[24] (This paper also cites useful references on animal research into the teratogenic effects of lead.) Multi-element studies involving lead are discussed below.

The relationship between lead exposure *in utero* and congenital abnormalities has already been mentioned. (See above.) Needleman and his colleagues have found it to be associated 'in a dose-related fashion with an increased risk for minor anomalies'.[25]

Prenatal exposure can result in lead intoxication in the newborn. In one report, an infant exposed in the eighth month *in utero* was delivered normally and found to have no detectable neurologic abnormality. However, testing at the age of 13 months showed she was functioning cognitively at the level of an 8–12-month child.[26] Another study measured the level of lead in umbilical cord blood at birth. Subsequent mental developmental testing at the ages of 6 months and 12 months showed that the higher the level of lead the lower the test scores. At neither age were scores related to current blood lead levels. The researchers concluded: 'Prenatal exposure to lead levels relatively common among urban populations appear to be associated with less favourable development through the first year of life.'[27] A further study by the same researcher, which concerned 'Longitudinal analyses of prenatal and postnatal lead exposure and early cognitive development', concluded that: 'It appears that the fetus may be adversely affected at blood lead concentrations well below 25 ug/dl, the level currently defined by the Center for Disease Control as the highest acceptable level for young children'.[28]

Research by Drs McConnell and Berry of the University of Birmingham gives us a clue as to why this should happen. They found that in rats lead tends to derange the development of the brain in a special way. If you think of the brain as a computer, then at birth, although all the parts are there, they have not all been connected. This happens over childhood, with the greater number being 'wired up' in early infancy. The lead stopped much of the 'wiring' and may well have meant some wrong connections being made. Other studies have shown that other parts of the brain closely involved with learning processes are also susceptible to damage by lead.[29]

Animal research with monkeys has confirmed that learning abilities are affected. In one study, monkeys in their first year of life showed no physical signs of toxicity, but all the lead-treated ones showed performance deficits on reversal learning tasks. The effects are not the result of delayed maturation, as the researchers report that '... Data currently being collected in this laboratory indicate that the deficit can be observed at least three years beyond final lead dosing. It therefore appears likely that this deficit represents a relatively permanent characteristic of the chronically lead-poisoned monkey'.[30]

The most widely quoted study on the effects of lead on children is that done by Needleman and his colleagues. They showed that at levels below those which were considered to produce symptoms of toxicity, the performance of children in the classroom was adversely affected. A wide range of behaviours was examined, including distractibility, persistence, dependence, organisational ability, hyperactivity, impulsiveness, frustration, day dreaming, ability to follow, and overall functioning, and it was found the higher the lead level, the poorer the performance in every measure.[31] Other studies have also indicated the negative effects of lead on learning abilities and classroom behaviour.[32-35]

Decreased hand-eye coordination and shortened reaction times, as well as physical effects, were seen in 45 adolescents and young adults with hair levels considered to be normal, with problems starting at levels as low as 10 ppm (parts per million). Most laboratories class up to 15 ppm as 'normal'.[36] (What this may mean for the acquisition of practical job skills and driving abilities has yet to be considered!)

A number of other studies have also suggested a link between hyperactivity and raised lead levels.[37,38] One looked at 13 children with no apparent cause for their hyperactivity and found that their behaviour improved when the lead was removed with lead-chelating medication.[39] A Danish study linked high levels with minimal cerebral dysfunction (MCD) – learning disabilities are often linked with hyperactivity or MCD.[40]

Cadmium

Cadmium is now a common pollutant which is highly dangerous to man as it accumulates in the kidneys and liver slowly, unless nutritional measures are taken to remove it or reduce absorption. It particularly builds up in people deficient of Vitamins C, D, B6, zinc, manganese, copper, selenium and/or calcium.[41] The main sources are cigarette smoking and processed foods, since in the refining of flour, the zinc in the germ and bran layers is removed leaving a high cadmium to zinc ratio. It is found in water, especially where impure zinc has been used in galvanising of the mains and pipes, through which soft water flows.[42] It is also widely used in manufacturing industries, including those concerned with paint, batteries, television sets and fertilisers.[43] It also comes from shellfish from polluted waters and galvanised containers[44] and coal burning.[45]

It is known to be embryotoxic in animals. Cleft palate and/or lip, other facial malformations and limb defects have been reported in a number of species.[46] Testicular and ovarian necrosis, and renal disorders are also found.[47] It has been found to impair reproduction in mice.[48] Cadmium accumulates in the placenta, causing placental necrosis if large amounts are given.[49] It also crosses the placenta.[50] Pregnant animals have developed toxaemia, an observation which has led one expert to wonder if 'one might suspect that toxaemia in humans may be due to excess cadmium and/or a lack of the nutrients that counteract the effect of cadmium'.[51]

In humans it has been associated with proteinuria[52] (protein in the urine) as well as low birth weight and small head circumference. (See below.)

The importance of zinc in counteracting the effects of cadmium has been demonstrated in animal research on the effects of cadmium on the testes. Pretreatment with zinc can abolish some of the adverse effects, though it does not reverse others.[53] When cadmium is injected subcutaneously into female rats it produces marked changes in the ovaries, the adverse effects initially increasing over time, although the ovaries do return to normal eventually.[54]

Mercury

Mercury has long been recognised as a poison. The 'Mad Hatter' of *Alice in Wonderland* was often a reality, as mercury was widely used in the millinery trade. The damage it can cause to the fetus was highlighted in the Japanese tragedy of Minamata, in which 23 children were born with cerebral palsy-like symptoms, varying from mild spasticity to severe mental retardation, blindness, chronic seizures and death.[55,56] Their mothers, free from symptoms themselves, had been exposed to mercury while pregnant. Mercury is readily passed through the placenta and fetal blood often contains concentrations 20 per cent greater than the maternal blood. Fetal brain tissue may be four times higher than the mother's brain tissue.[57] Adults and older children were also affected, with a total of 46 dying.

There are three basic forms, elemental, non-organic and organic. The elemental and non-organic forms tend to be slowly absorbed and readily excreted, unlike the organic forms, which are easily absorbed and slow to be eliminated. Thus, the main dangers lie in the latter, especially methyl mercury, although there are conditions linked to elemental mercury. These include psychological disturbances, oral cavity disorders, gastro-intestinal, cardiovascular, neurologic, respiratory, immunological and endocrine effects. In severe cases there are hallucinations and manic-depression. Organic mercury exposure is linked with psychological symptoms which develop into paralysis, vision, speech and hearing problems, loss of memory, uncoordination, renal damage and general central nervous system dysfunctions. Eventually coma and death can occur.[58]

Metallic mercury vapour has been reported to affect men exposed to it in a serious way for prospective parents. In one study of nine men exposed after an accident, all complained of a loss of libido, lasting in some cases up to eight years. One reported temporary impotence for 18 months.[59]

Animal work by Dr Joan Spyker suggests that the adverse effects may be long-term. Mice exposed *in utero* did not appear outwardly different from controls until they were about 18 months old (middle-aged). The experimental mice then contracted severe infections, implying an immune system impaired prenatally. They lost all pretence of normalcy, aging quickly and prematurely. Only extensive investigation, magnifying the brain tissues 48,000 times, showed slight damage to the individual cells – yet this slight damage was responsible for their problems. Dr Spyker points out that the victims of Minamata are deteriorating just as the animal model predicted.[60]

The main sources of mercury are pesticides and fungicides (see Chapter 11), fish, industrial processes and dental fillings. The larger the fish, the greater the concentration, with tuna fish being the most likely source in the UK.[61] Freshwater fish can also be contaminated if the river has been polluted by factory effluent, or water run off fields which have been subjected to mercury-containing agrochemicals. It is found in slimicides, used in paper-manufacture to stop the growth of slime moulds.[62] If your hair level is high, it would be wise to have your water checked.

The major current controversy around the dangers of mercury concerns mercury-containing amalgams used in dentistry.[63,64] Dentists have been aware of mercury poisoning for many years – indeed, 147 years ago the American Society of Dental Surgeons was opposed to such amalgams. (They were overruled by their members, many of whom must later on have suffered from toxic effects!)[65] Sweden has now banned mercury in dental work on pregnant women as a prelude to a total ban.

It appears that some large marine mammals ingest high levels of selenium which detoxifies mercury, especially if taken with Vitamin E.[66]

Aluminium

Aluminium is easily absorbed, accumulating in the arteries. It is now linked with Alzheimer's Disease, though scientists are quick to point out that there is no conclusive proof. However, it is known that aluminium can destroy many vitamins as it readily binds with other substances. It weakens the lining of the gut. It inhibits fluorine and phosphorus metabolism, resulting in mineral loss from the bones over a long period. Excessive amounts can lead to constipation, colic, excessive perspiration, loss of appetite, nausea, skin problems and fatigue. Adverse effects associated with the body's attempts to clear itself, in which aluminium salts are found in small quantities in the blood, include paralysis and areas of numbness, with fatty degeneration of the kidney and liver, as well as symptoms of gastrointestinal inflammation.[67] Thus, it can seriously compromise nutritional status. It has been linked with kidney problems in babies, with the researchers concluding that formula feed should be aluminium-free for neonates and infants with reduced kidney function.[68] (Why not for all, we ask?) It has been associated with behavioural problems and autism.[69] Mice fed large doses had no symptoms, but the next three generations of offspring had growth defects.[70]

The major sources include antacids, antiperspirants and food additives, especially an anti-caking agent found in milk substitutes.[71,72] In some places, aluminium flocculents are added to the water, so you should have your water tested at the tap if your hair level is high. Aluminium saucepans and other cooking utensils impart some metal if they are in contact with the food. Leaf vegetables, rhubarb, apple and other acid fruits are especially problematic. Pressure cookers are worse than ordinary pans. Kettles and aluminium teapots are potent sources, particularly if the tea is allowed to stand for a long time. Work at University College, Cardiff, suggests that our major food source of aluminium is tea, since the tea plant thrives on alum soils, so it is fed with alum. (Think of all that tea drunk in psychiatric hospitals!) Foil-wrapped foods, such as meats, fish, poultry, and pies made in foil saucers, are other sources. Foil-wrapped fats and acid foods are the worst.

Copper

The contraceptive pill and copper coil can both cause copper levels in the body to rise. (See Chapter 9.) Excess levels may be embryotoxic or teratogenic.[73] They are certainly known to produce behavioural symptoms, such as uncontrollable rages,[74] and are linked with toxaemia.[75] Copper levels rise naturally during pregnancy, so if a woman conceives with a raised level she is at risk of overloading her body. This could lead to postpartum depression.[76] Raised levels are associated with low levels of zinc and manganese, both of which are known to cause birth defects. (See Chapter 5.)

Other sources of copper may be the drinking water in areas where the water is soft and acid, or where it has been heated through an Ascot heater. Always fill the kettle from the cold tap. If you have been using a filter for two weeks and seen the white contents of the filter change to blueish green, you have a significant amount of copper in your water. You should continue to filter, changing the cartridge regularly.

Copper kettles, pans and jewellery are also sources. There may be external contamination of hair from Henna dyes and rinses, and from swimming-pool water where the pool has been treated with a copper-containing algicide. For an accurate reading, you should cease the contamination for six weeks before having another hair mineral analysis.

Other metals

Animal tests have brought arsenic, lithium and selenium under suspicion as embryotoxic or teratogenic.[77] Arsenic has also been found to act as a transplacental carcinogen.[78] A study among workers in Sweden has implicated arsenic in decreased birth weight and an increased rate of spontaneous abortion, but the design of the study was poor so the results are subject to debate. Depending on when it is administered it is said it can cause neural tube defects, agenesis and renal problems.[79]

Multi-element studies

As far back as 1969, it was reported that 'Cadmium teratogenicity is dramatically augmented by lead when they are administered concurrently'.[80] Lead and cadmium often occur together. Their concentrations in hair and blood show strong positive correlations and their overt symptoms of toxicity are not unalike. These similarities have led some researchers to the view that 'It is possible that some of the deleterious effects attributed to lead in correlational studies may instead be due to cadmium'.[81] They conducted a study on hair cadmium and lead levels in relation to cognitive functioning in children, in which the results showed that hair cadmium and lead were significantly correlated with intelligence tests and school achievement, but not with motor impairment scores. Statistical analysis suggested that 'cadmium has a stronger effect on verbal IQ than does lead and that lead has a stronger effect on performance IQ than does cadmium'.[82]

A few years before this, Professor Bryce-Smith and his colleagues, aware of the inadequacies of single element studies, had reviewed the levels of four elements: lead, cadmium, zinc and calcium in stillbirths' bones and cartilage. They found that cadmium concentrates in the stillbirths were ten times greater than the levels normally found in human bone. Lead levels were also raised. Low calcium and zinc were sometimes associated with these marked elevations.[83] (See also lead above for reference to this study.)

Given the results of these, and many other studies, showing that lead and cadmium can have adverse effects on the fetus and older children, could they also cause problems for the neonate? Research has shown they do!

Spurred on by the results of the four element study, a much larger project was done by Professor Bryce-Smith and his colleagues. This major study has taken a number of years to complete, revealing much of interest throughout. In an interim report in 1981, Professor Bryce-Smith said that for all the elements being studied (at that time, 36), the levels of fetal and maternal blood were about the same. Only in lead levels was there a difference, with the fetal level about 95 per cent of the maternal. He went on to explain the significance of this: 'This means that the placenta passes all elements, both nutrients and toxins, to the fetus from the maternal circulation with little or no selectivity or filtering defect. We can see no evidence for a significant barrier to protect the fetus from inorganic toxins such as mercury, arsenic, and antimony; and there is only a slight, but significant ($p=0.01$) barrier in the case of lead for normal births only.'[84] Having begun by analysing nine tissues, including maternal and fetal (umbilical) cord whole blood and serum, amniotic fluid, placenta, and scalp hair from the mother and neonate, later on they decided that the placental element levels showed the clearest correlations with indices of fetal development for supposedly 'normal' births. Thus it was with this tissue that they continued the investigation.

In the first written report on the final 37 elements studied, the researchers observed highly significant negative relationships between placental cadmium and lead levels, and birth weight, head circumference and placental weight. The smaller the birth weight, head circumference and placental weight was, the higher the level of cadmium and lead. There was a statistically significant positive correlation between placental cadmium and lead levels where birth weights were less than 3,000 g. For higher birth weights, the correlation, though still positive, was not significant. Placental zinc showed significant positive relationships with birth weights up to 3,000 g and head circumference of less than 34 cm, i.e. the lower the zinc level, the lower the birth weight and the smaller the head circumference.

With respect to other elements, there was 'a weak positive correlation between placental iron and head circumference, and stronger but negative correlations for chlorine, vanadium, and lanthanum'. However, placental levels of iron did not correlate with birth weight, nor were the iron levels or birth weights significantly raised in those mothers receiving iron supplements. Indeed, the results in iron and zinc led the researchers to suggest that more emphasis should be paid to zinc supplements than to iron.

The final point made in the paper states that 'In cases of cadmium, lead and zinc, biological, neurobehavioural, and biosocial studies in which the levels of all three elements are measured may prove more informative than those involving single elements'.[85]

Much the same conclusion was reached by the researchers who conducted further investigations into lead, cadmium and cognitive functioning. Looking at the protective effects of zinc and calcium against toxic metals, they found that higher zinc levels seemed to protect against the effects of cadmium, while calcium did the same against lead. They concluded: 'The results suggest that the effects of heavy metal pollutants on cognitive function cannot adequately be assessed without concurrently evaluating the status of essential nutrients with which these toxins are known to interact metabolically.'[86]

Detoxifying the body
The preferred method of detoxification must, undoubtedly, be nutritional, since it does not have the same potential for adverse side effects as drugs. (There is a drug called EDTA which can be used in acute poisoning, though it is not to be recommended.) It binds the elements to it so they are removed from the body along with the EDTA. However, it removes essential minerals as well, so the doctor needs to check to see you are not short of calcium, magnesium and other nutrients. Alternatively, penicillamine may be given. The following is a guide to the nutrients and foods that are helpful in removing toxic metals.

Vitamin C and zinc supplements were used successfully in reducing blood lead levels of psychiatric outpatients in one study. The treatment was also found to lower blood copper levels. Subjects included some hyperactive children.[87] Vitamin C has also been shown to lower cadmium levels in birds.[88]

Calcium helps prevent absorption, as well as removing lead from the tissues. Vitamin D is necessary for calcium metabolism and to help displace lead from the bones. Vitamin B1, taken with a B-Complex, provides protection against lead damage. Lecithin can also help in protection, while Vitamin A helps to activate the enzymes needed for detoxification. Trace elements, in addition to zinc, which are protective include chromium and manganese. Garlimac tablets are often used but they need to be combined with manganese to preserve the levels of manganese. In the diet, peas, lentils and beans act as detoxifiers. Algin, found in seaweeds, attracts lead to it in the gut and carries it out of the body. Yoghourt, garlic, onions, bananas and fruits such as apples and pears which contain pectin (especially the pips) help to reduce absorption, as well as detoxifying.[89] Vitamin E may also reduce lead poisoning.[90] Manganese and selenium are also useful in detoxification.

It has also been found that sunlight can help remove toxic metals in animal studies.[91]

○ CHECKLIST FOR REDUCING TOXIC METAL LEVELS IN THE BODY.
1. Eat nutritious food and supplement your diet wisely. Include many of the foods mentioned in the section on detoxification above.

2. Wash foods carefully – a vinegar solution of 1 tablespoonful to a pint of water will remove much surface lead, but be careful not to soak, as the essential nutrients will be lost to the water.
3. Avoid unlined tinned foods especially, though you are best avoiding all tins. If the label on the tin does not specify it is lined, you will have to check on opening.
4. Buy organic foods.
5. If you buy food which contains additives, read the labels and check the additives in the Foresight booklet *Find Out*.
6. Avoid aluminium kitchenware, foil and foods containing aluminium additives.
7. Have your water tested for toxic metals. Use a filter, being sure that you follow the manufacturer's instructions.
8. Avoid, where possible, heavily polluted air, e.g. do not stand around unnecessarily in heavy traffic. Close car windows in tunnels. Fit net curtains to windows facing a busy road and wash frequently.
9. Check labels of toiletries and cosmetics. Be especially wary of deodorants and anti-perspirants, unless they specify the ingredients.
10. Refuse mercury-containing dental fillings.
11. Check what chemicals you may be exposed to in the course of your work. Ask about safety precautions and obey the rules.

CHAPTER 8

Problems in the Twentieth Century: Drugs

INFORMATION ON HOW TO KEEP YOUR BABY SAFE FROM UNNECESSARY DRUGS — AND WHY YOU NEED TO DO SO.

In discussing drugs we often ignore those which are socially acceptable. Yet if we take these into account it is sadly no exaggeration to say that we are a nation of drug addicts, hooked on tea, coffee, Coca-Cola, cigarettes, alcohol, aspirins and other drugs bought over the counter, not to mention those prescribed by doctors, and those banned by law. *ALL* drugs have side effects and in prescribing, a doctor should consciously, and conscientiously, weigh these against the benefits. We should also do the same for other drugs, keeping a balance. A number of books and articles are available to help.[1,2,3] This chapter outlines what we know about the effects of drugs on fertility, pregnancy and lactation. (We omit the pill, as this is discussed in the next chapter.)

Factors common to all drugs

It does not matter what the drug is: it will always have an effect on the body's biochemistry, which is not natural. Reviewing the literature on how drugs and chemicals adversely affect the offspring of male mammals, Dr Justin Joffe, Professor of Psychology, University of Vermont, concluded that, regardless of the species of the animal, the chemical given, its dose, and its timing, there were three main effects which seemed common to many studies: smaller litters, lower birth weights in those animals actually born, and higher mortality rates in the newborn.[4] During pregnancy, it is now recognised that the placenta does *not* act as a barrier, across which toxins do not pass. Substances, as the Thalidomide and DES tragedies showed, can reach the fetus with devastating consequences, although there may be some ways in which protection is offered by the mother. (Thalidomide, a drug given to prevent morning sickness, caused limb deformities in many children. Di-Ethyl Stilbestrol, another drug given to prevent miscarriage, resulted in cancer in the reproductive organs of the children at puberty.) Drugs can also reach the baby through the mother's milk.[5,6,7,8]

Although there are compulsory tests which drugs have to pass before going into use, there is doubt over the effectiveness of the tests. At least one statistician has claimed that the basic test method may give the wrong result in 50 per cent of tests.[9] Moreover, the tests do not always consider synergistic effects of taking two or more substances simultaneously. The dangers to the user of mixing alcohol and sleeping tablets are well known, but the dangers to the fetus of most combinations of drugs are not usually discussed. Adverse reactions are sometimes magnified when two or more substances are taken together, though this will depend on a number of factors, including the drugs themselves.[10] Babies born to mothers who smoke marihuana and drink alcohol have been found to have a greater risk of fetal alcohol syndrome (see below).[11] They are at greater risk of low birth weight if both cigarettes and marihuana are smoked.[12] Caffeine-cigarette interactions have also been associated with low birth weight.[13] Some of the effects are indicated in the drug information, which will list contraindications. This is why it is so important for the doctor to be aware of ALL drugs either prospective parent or pregnant woman is taking.

We have placed great emphasis in this book on nutrition, and it is due to their effects in this area that drugs are probably at their most detrimental. Drugs affect nutrients, such as vitamins and minerals, in a number of ways. They can lead to impaired absorption, as, for example, when laxatives form a physical barrier to fats by dissolving them before the body can ingest them. Others, such as mineral oil, may absorb essential nutrients which are then excreted. They may compete with nutrients at the gut wall, and the nutrients may lose the fight! They can cause increased excretion of nutrients that the body needs. Alcohol is a classic example of this, causing excretion of a number of nutrients, including some B vitamins, zinc and magnesium. Yet others may lead to increased requirements of certain nutrients, or cause redistribution of nutrients in the body at the cellular level. They may even decrease nutrient requirement, as in the case of the Pill and iron. To add to the complexity of all this, they may do a number of these together![14]

We shall now take a closer look at different types of drugs and their effects on the fetus and pregnancy, starting with prescribed drugs and those bought over the counter, before looking at the 'social poisons'. We are deliberately leaving the illegal street drugs to last, because while they have devastating effects as we shall see, they are only taken by a minority and pose comparatively fewer problems for most prospective parents.

Prescribed and self-prescribed drugs

Ideally, both parents should not be taking any drugs prior to conception, and the female should not take any during pregnancy or breastfeeding, but this is not always possible.

○ TREATMENT FOR DIABETES OR EPILEPSY. Where drugs are considered necessary, as in diabetes or epilepsy, for example, the doctor should be sure he is fully informed of drug-nutrient interactions and should make whatever recommendations he can to minimise the adverse effects. (We should mention, though, that many people with these conditions find they do not need drugs when their deficiency and allergy problems have been fully resolved on the Foresight programme.) Many food additives and pesticides have been implicated in the causation of epilepsy. (See Chapter 11.) Clearly a balance needs to be struck, and a drug may be preferable to the risk of a stillbirth or deformity. But it is often possible to treat a condition using nutritional methods or complementary methods, such as relaxation training, rather than risk a drug.

It is likely that the teratogenicity (capability of causing damage to the fetus) of drugs is frequently related to the drug/nutrient interactions mentioned above. It has been suggested that the Thalidomide tragedy may have been due to riboflavin (Vitamin B2) deficiency.[15] In experimental animals, this deficiency produces malformations like those suffered by the Thalidomide victims. Thalidomide resembles riboflavin in chemical structure and could therefore have blocked the uptake of the vitamin.

○ ANTI-CONVULSANTS. Anti-convulsant drugs, especially dilantin and phenobarbitone, induce biochemical evidence of folate (folic acid) deficiency if the diet contains a barely adequate amount of the vitamin. With evidence that pregnant women on anti-convulsants have an increased likelihood of having a malformed baby, it would seem wise to supplement their diets with folate. However, care must be taken to ensure a dose of the drug high enough to be effective clinically, as the additional folate may make the drug less effective at the original dose. The work by Labadorios with rats supports this view.[16] These drugs also increase the requirement for Vitamin D. A deficiency of Vitamin D is dangerous during pregnancy, and in the child who is being breastfed there could be a risk of rickets.

○ ANTI-DEPRESSANTS. Anti-depressants which are monoaminase blockers are known to decrease sperm count and motility.[17,18] Tricyclic anti-depressants do not have the same effects.

○ ASPIRIN. Claims about an association between aspirin-taking, low birth weight and a high perinatal mortality rate have come from Australia.[19,20] Their findings were not confirmed in two US studies, although the subjects were taking smaller doses.[21,22] A study looking at aspirin use and subsequent child IQ and ability to concentrate found that use in the first half of pregnancy was significantly related to a lower IQ and inability to concentrate in those children who had been exposed to aspirin in the womb.[23] (Under a Foresight clinician, the source of the pain would be located and the problem treated in advance of the pregnancy.) It is therefore very worrying that the Medical Research Council should be considering a trial using aspirin to lessen the risk of pre-eclampsia.[24]

○ TRANQUILLISERS AND SLEEPING PILLS. Benzodiazepines, which are often prescribed as tranquillisers, should be avoided at any time during pregnancy. They have been linked with visible malformations, functional deficits, and behavioural problems in exposed children. They can disturb the central nervous system, which includes the brain, in the very early stages of pregnancy.[25] Other researchers have suggested that mothers who take them during the first three months of pregnancy are 3.3 times more likely to have a baby with an oral cleft (hare lip and/or cleft palate).[26] In many cases, tranquillisers are taken to counteract the effects of overstimulation by other social drugs (such as excessive coffee) or the effects of deficiencies such as zinc and magnesium.

○ HORMONES. Sex hormones used therapeutically in pregnancy may cause malformation of the fetal sex organs, as well as aberrant behaviour. Taken during delivery, they may affect the neonate's weight gain and response to nursing.[27]

○ BETA-BLOCKERS. Research has also shown that the male is not immune to side effects of drugs which may interfere with his fertility.[28,29] Phelezine, a beta-blocker, decreases sperm count and motility.[30,31]

○ SMOKING. The dangers to health of smoking are still the subject of much debate, but there can be no dispute that smoking during pregnancy is a major cause of abnormal pregnancies, avoidable illness, handicap and deformity in children.[32] Babies born to smoking mothers are, on average, 7 ounces lighter than those born to non-smoking mothers, though this weight reduction may not be significant.[33] Richmond, however, found that women who smoke double their risk of having a low birth-weight baby.[34] The reduction in growth is mostly due to hypoxia, but nicotine itself causes decreases in uterine blood flow and placental amino acid uptake.[35] In a study of 50,000 pregnancies, Naeye[36] reported abnormally large areas of dead tissue in the placentas of both smoking mothers and women who had smoked in the past. Such damage to the placenta interferes with the nutrition of the fetus. Cadmium, an inorganic poison present in smoke, becomes concentrated in the placenta[37] (see Chapter 7), while cyanide, also present as a result of the hypertensive effect of thiocyanate, interferes with fetal nutrition, impeding growth and leading to low birth weight.[38] Heavy smokers and drinkers have a six times greater risk of stillbirth.[39] Heavy smokers also have a higher risk of spontaneous abortions and fetal malformations, including cleft palate, hare lip, and central nervous system abnormalities.[40] There is a higher incidence of premature births[41] and short-for-date full-term infants in smokers.[42] There seems to be a greater risk of tubal pregnancy for current smokers, compared with women who have never smoked.[43] It is possible that minor brain damage may be caused. Studies have shown poorer learning abilities in children born to smokers, compared with those born to non-smokers.[44]

All this is not surprising if you remember that there are over 4,000 compounds in tobacco smoke. Nicotine is the most widely known and is the addictive substance. Besides the effects already mentioned, it has been shown to lower hormone levels in animals, which may affect fertility and milk production.[45] It also interferes with nutrient absorption in the fetus. Nor are passive smokers free from risk to their fetus, especially if they are in smoky atmospheres for long periods. Carbon monoxide, released by burning cigarettes and cigars, builds up in the atmosphere. High levels lead to a reduction in the oxygen-carrying capacity of the blood, depriving the fetus of an optimum level of oxygen.

The effects of male smoking can be serious. German workers have reported that the fetus can be affected by the amount the father smokes. Where he smoked heavily, the child was more than two-and-a-half times more likely to have malformations. Facial malformations were related to the smoking level in the man.[46] Smoking lowers testosterone levels, and affects spermatogenesis, sperm morphology and sperm motility.[47]

Children of smokers have higher rates of illness, particularly respiratory infections, and increased risk of cot deaths. Intellectual, physical and emotional development is slower than in children of non-smokers.[48]

Although there is not yet agreement among experts, some are suggesting the existence of a fetal tobacco syndrome. They claim there are certain features common to children born of heavy smokers.[49] Smoking is known to cause changes in the appearance of adults, and in a study of the appearance of newborn infants, medical and nursing students were able to distinguish correctly, in significant numbers, between those born to smoking and non-smoking mothers based on intuitive selection.[50]

Caffeine

'The sufferer is tremulous and loses his self-command; he is subject to fits of agitation and depression; he loses colour and has a haggard appearance. The appetite falls off, and symptoms of gastric catarrh may be manifested. The heart also suffers; it palpates, or it intermits. As with other such agents, a renewed dose of the poison gives temporary relief, but at the cost of future misery.'[51]

So wrote the authors of a 1906 medical textbook when they described the caffeine addict.

Found in tea, coffee, cocoa, soft drinks, foods and medicines, caffeine is a widely used alkaloid drug, which has an initial stimulating effect in small doses. However, although it can temporarily relieve fatigue, it also raises blood pressure and stimulates the kidneys, in addition to the effects mentioned above. Five or more cups a day is what it is reckoned you have to drink to become addicted, though this does not mean that everyone drinking this amount will be an addict.[52] Most people will have more than this amount in their daily food and drink, unless they check their foods and drinks carefully.

Most research on its effects on both male and female reproduction systems is not encouraging. In certain amounts, it can affect sperm motility,[52] with large amounts causing complete immobilisation.[53] Consumption during pregnancy has been associated with abortion, chromosomal abnormality and congenital multi-abnormality,[54] and late spontaneous abortion.[55]

Since it appears in so many foods and beverages, the only way you can be sure of avoiding it, or controlling your intake, is to buy fresh foods and do your own baking and watch the ingredients. Decaffeinated is not recommended, as it contains other stimulants, and possibly harmful residues, such as pesticides.[56]

Alcohol

It is now accepted that alcohol during pregnancy may have serious consequences for the fetus. There seems to be no dispute, for example, on the existence of fetal alcohol syndrome. However, there are still mixed messages about how much alcohol it is safe to drink.[57] Be advised by an expert on early embryology, Professor Matthew Kaufman. Explaining that it is impossible to advise on a safe limit he added that, 'the only thing we can say is safe is none at all until child-bearing is over, though presumably that would be totally unacceptable socially'.[58] He is probably right, so the Foresight message is: *NO alcohol in the preconception preparation phase for both partners, and during pregnancy for the woman.*

Alcohol travels through the blood stream to affect the sperm, egg and fetus. One animal study gave male mice alcohol for 26 days then sobered them up for two days before breeding. The litters produced were only half the normal number of pups, and only 12 per cent of them survived for more than a month.[59] Kaufman has found that serious chromosome faults appear in up to 20 per cent of mice embryos after only moderate doses of dilute alcohol. He believes that, since alcohol has a specific effect on the chromosomes, ingestion is one of the major factors in thousands of miscarriages, as well as in many of the babies born with mental and physical handicaps.[60]

Male drinking habits are often overlooked, yet this acceptable social drug is known to affect the sperm. In heavy drinkers, the sperm often lack normal tails, which will affect sperm motility.[61] Two researchers were able to predict, statistically, a decrease of about 4¾ ounces (137 grams) in infant birth weight if the father had an average of two drinks or more daily, or at least five on one occasion in the month leading up to conception.[62] Russian research has also suggested sperm abnormalities in alcoholic fathers can cause fetal abnormalities.[63]

The Maternity Alliance has published a useful review, written by the Wynns, of research on the damage caused, such as higher spontaneous abortion rates, more stillbirths, reduced fertility and more abnormalities.[64]

1. Central nervous dysfunction, with mental retardation of varying degree. In some children IQ may be low, although in others it may be average, but they may have learning problems, such as a poor attention span.
2. Growth deficiencies, being of low birth weight, and short in length at birth. Normal post-natal growth does not happen.
3. Facial abnormalities, with distinct features, including low nose bridge, narrow upper lip, small chin and a flat face.
4. Other malformations, especially heart and dental defects.

It is also suggested that there may be hyperactivity, distractibility and short attention span.[65] Other researchers refer to defects of the mouth, genito-urinary system, hernias and birthmarks, as well as a weak ability to suck.[66] Where a number of these are found in the same child, he/she may be identified as a victim of fetal alcohol syndrome.

The Fetal Alcohol Study Group drew up a set of minimal criteria for diagnosis of this syndrome, covering specific aspects of growth, the central nervous system and characteristic head and facial features.[67] It is difficult to assess the incidence of the syndrome, since definitions vary. Some say 0.4 to 3.1 per live births, but others say it may range as high as 78–690 per 1,000 live births in alcoholic mothers. If one includes the partial syndrome or infants suffering from other effects, it could be from 1.7 to 90.1 per 1,000 depending on definition. What seems certain is that the condition is irreversible after birth.[68]

Marijuana – pot, cannabis

It is often claimed that marijuana smoking is safer than cigarette smoking: the truth is that both have serious adverse effects on health. Research, however, is suggesting that marijuana is four times more dangerous because the smoker takes deeper breaths and holds the breath for longer.[69] This results in three times more tar in the lungs and five times more carbon monoxide.

The psychoactive substance in marijuana is called tetrahydrocannabinol (THC), which has the steroid structure found in the sex hormones and in certain hormones of the adrenal gland. THC tends to accumulate in the ovaries and testes. In women it upsets the menstrual cycle, though it is possible to become tolerant to it, in which case the cycle is restored.[70] In men, heavy use of five to 18 joints a week for six months has been noted to cause a marked lowering of blood testosterone, lower sperm count, greater than usual impotency and diminished libido.[71] Sperm motility is also affected and there is an increase in the number of abnormal sperm.[72]

The drug has been shown to affect the synthesis of DNA, and to slow the growth rate of cells.[73] In animals, it has been linked with an increase in fetal deaths and malformations.[74] In humans, it is likely that babies will be smaller because of the increased carbon monoxide levels, which will make less oxygen available to the fetus. It induces chromosome damage.[75] There seem to be dose-related behavioural effects, which occur in all babies born to mothers who are heavy abusers. Prolonged or arrested labour may occur.[76]

Cocaine
Cocaine use has increased dramatically in the UK and the USA in the last decade. Animal studies have reported that it is teratogenic in mice even at non-toxic doses.[77] Rats showed higher resorption rates and a significantly lower fetal weight.[78] In a study of three groups of women, 50 cocaine only abusers, 110 multi-drug abusers, and 340 non-abusers concluded that 'Cocaine abuse in humans significantly reduces the weight of the fetus, increases the stillbirth rate related to *abrupto placentae*, and is associated with a higher malformation rate'. The babies suffered mild withdrawal symptoms.[79]

Heroin
Heroin belongs to a group of drugs derived from the opium plants. Other opiate narcotics include opium, morphine and codeine. They are all very addictive, heroin especially, and are known to lead to decreased fertility and atrophy of the male accessory sex organs. They also decrease testosterone.[80]

In women addicts, there are many complications during pregnancy. Such women have a three times greater risk of stillbirth than non-addicts, a four times greater risk of prematurity, and a six times greater chance of a baby who has suffered growth deficiency. A significantly higher number of infants with congenital abnormalities can be seen. There are also higher rates of jaundice, and respiratory distress syndrome. Low birth weight and small size for gestational age are found. There is increased perinatal mortality, with rates up to 37 per cent in some studies.[81] Other fetal complications noted include infections and episodes of stress.[82] There may be long-term effects on growth and behaviour, with regard to perceptual and organising abilities.[83] The babies are born addicted to the drug and have to undergo withdrawal, which is stressful even to adults, let alone the immature body of the neonate.

How to overcome addiction
There are no easy paths to overcoming addiction, be it to sugar, or heroin. It is doubtful if those people who quit smoking or drinking overnight, without a qualm, were ever 'addicted'. They may merely have had to give up a habit, though even this will not always be so simple. Nor is it true that addiction is a psychological condition – whatever the substance of abuse, the abuser will be in a state of biochemical or physiological imbalance which has probably provoked the addiction initially. However, there are steps that the individual can take to overcome his/her addiction without a difficult physical withdrawal. (These are described fully in *The Hidden Addiction*.[84] We would strongly urge anyone with a problem to read this book and share it with their doctor.)

> **Warning**
> Abrupt withdrawal from drugs during pregnancy may precipitate an abortion or premature labour.[85] (Of course, if you have followed the Foresight programme, you will not be pregnant while still addicted!)

Outline of treatment programme for overcoming addictions
1. Start at the beginning of your preconception care plan, at least five months before you plan to conceive, remembering that conception should not occur until you are both healthy.
2. Enlist your doctor's help. See you have a thorough check-up, with biochemical tests. Tell him if you feel depressed. Ask for a referral to a doctor trained in nutritional medicine.
3. Educate yourself about addiction generally and about your substance(s) of abuse.
4. Make a personal commitment to the treatment.
5. Abstain from taking the addicting substance.
6. Avoid new or substitute addictions. These include alcohol, sugar-foods, caffeine, and drugs, except those considered essential by your doctor. Sometimes alcoholics will be advised to drink coffee or eat sugar – this does not help you. It can even hinder progress, and will certainly not build better health, which is what you are trying to do. Your greatest incentive to staying off your addiction is feeling better without it, physically, mentally and emotionally.
7. Start a good nutritional plan. This is fundamental to your progress and to your improving health. (See Chapter 5.)
8. Detoxify your body with Vitamin C and other nutrients. Restore vitamin and mineral deficiencies and remove toxins using nutritional supplements, as advised by a doctor who is trained in nutritional medicine.
9. Take daily exercise. It will help your nutritional programme, as well as your general progress.
10. Find new and fulfilling activities.
11. Be positive! You are probably having to change quite a bit of your lifestyle, so start enjoying yourself. (Adapted from *The Hidden Addiction*.[86])

Checklist

Review the drugs you use.

Do you take:	Action to be taken if the answer is 'Yes':
Drugs prescribed by your doctor?	Continue to take the drugs until you have seen your doctor. Ask him/her why you need them. Is there a safe non-drug alternative treatment? What do you need

	to do to minimise the side effects, especially with reference to your nutritional status?
Alcohol?	Don't drink during preconception preparation (both partners), pregnancy and lactation (female).
Tobacco?	Don't at all! You risk harming your baby and, after the birth, you are harming your child if you smoke in the same environment (both partners).
Caffeine?	Reduce your intake by limiting the amount of tea and coffee you drink. Avoid colas and chocolate, not only because of the caffeine they contain, but also the sugar (both partners).
'Street' drugs?	Avoid! If you are addicted seek professional help and follow the programme outlined in this chapter (both partners).

CHAPTER 9

Problems in the Twentieth Century: Harmful Contraception Methods

HELP WITH RECOGNISING THE HAZARDS OF HORMONE MANIPULATION, AND WHY YOU NEED TO KNOW.

The Pill
It is probably true that no other drugs have received so much attention as the oral contraceptive pill (the 'Pill'). It is also probably true that the general public and much of the medical profession have never been so misled about a group of drugs. Even to the lay person, there are obvious discrepancies – for example, many gynaecologists seem unable to explain why steroids which are said to be unsafe for women over the age of 35 years are safe when women reach the menopause. Logic would suggest that the risks are at least the same, if not greater with increasing age. But what are these steroids and what are their risks? Are we really being deceived into believing they are safe?

What the pill is
Oral contraceptive pills generally contain two hormones (steroids), oestrogen and progestogen, in various combinations according to trade name (the combined pill). The mini-pill contains just progestogen, and can cause irregular bleeding and has a higher chance of pregnancy with its use. But it really does not matter which type a woman is taking, because it is the ingested or injected hormones that are said to be dangerous to women's health.

How the pills work
We saw in Chapter 6 how the levels of oestrogen and progesterone in your body rise and fall during the menstrual cycle, being high towards the end of the month. Both oestrogen and progesterone remain high throughout pregnancy, thereby preventing the ovaries

from preparing another egg to release. The combined pill works by confusing the body into thinking that it is pregnant, by keeping the hormone levels high. Because oestrogen alone caused irregular bleeding, a progestogen was added to the pill. The commonly prescribed mainly progestogen pills make the cervical mucus thick and sticky and the lining of the womb atrophied and thin. Both of these actions increase the contraceptive effects, making it difficult for the sperm to enter the womb or for the womb to accept a fertilised egg.

Normal menstruation is prevented – indeed, the pill is often prescribed for painful periods, on the assumption that it relieves them. What is often not understood by women is that it does so by stopping normal ovulatory cycles, including periods, altogether, substituting withdrawal bleeding for a normal period when the pill is stopped for a few days each month. Dr Ellen Grant maintains that painful cramps due to prostaglandin release may be part of a response to inflammation and using steroid hormones to suppress this natural response does nothing to treat the inflammation of the neck of the womb, if present.[1] (Foresight doctors find that in women of all ages, simple vitamin, mineral and essential oil supplements are a much safer way to relieve painful periods. They also carry no risk of interfering with the brain control of ovulation.)

'Lies, damned lies and statistics', not to mention studies on the pill!
From all the information available, one can expect that doctors will pay serious heed to reports issued by one of their own professional colleges. The Royal College of General Practitioners' Oral Contraceptive Study was one of two large scale trials started in 1968.[2] It is best regarded not as a clinical trial but 'as a record of the natural history of two cohorts of women, one of which has used oral contraceptives while the other has not'.[3] Unfortunately, it has erroneously been accorded the status of a proper trial, with the interim report being quoted in the press as suggesting that the pill is a safe drug. Yet when one examines the report closely, there can be no conclusion other than one which points to the pill as a dangerous drug on the data available to date, without considering what damage could be inflicted in the long term. Unfortunately, since the 1974 Report, there has not been a comprehensive follow-up.

(Dr Ellen Grant has written a critique of the work in her book, *The Bitter Pill*.[4] With her consent we draw on it in the following paragraphs.)

47,174 women were enrolled on the study during 1968 and 1969. Even from the start, the control and experimental groups were not randomised nor equivalent. Obviously, the experimental (pill-taking) group did not contain women in whom illness had already rendered the pill inadvisable, so this group was likely to be healthier than the controls. The drop-out rate from the pill-users group was large, even in the first three years: by 1979, it was enormous, with only a small percentage of the original pill-users group still taking the pill. The researchers had even switched 6,000 women in the control group to the pill-users (experimental) group to boost numbers. Why had so many dropped out?

Dr Grant believes that the 'big exodus was hardly surprising as the 1974 report showed a large number of medical conditions were increased in pill users...an increase in over sixty conditions.[5] She presents evidence to show the increase in many of these, for example, in suicide, cancer and vascular conditions. Dr Grant's detailed review to the *British Medical Journal*, complaining that 'the high drop-out and side-effects rates did not justify further use of the pill', was cut to a short letter.[6]

Nor did the study measure 'total morbidity', as was claimed. It measured conditions that the doctors recognised – there are a number of important conditions that many doctors do not always acknowledge, such as some allergies and widespread nutritional deficiencies.

Dr Grant is not alone in her concern. As far back as 1974, a lay person's guide to better health[7] gave an overview of the dangers of the pill, including quotes from eminent doctors to a Congressional subcommittee and from H. Williams' book, published in 1969, in which he said: 'In fact, the pill has been shown to be capable of affecting any or all systems and organs in the body, with a great variety of consequences.'[8] In the same year, Barbara Seamans wrote: 'Very few pill-users have the slightest notion of the potency of the drugs they are ingesting, or how the little pills may affect their own health or their still unborn children.'[9]

The risks associated with the pill
There are many risks to health associated with the pill. Dr Paavo Airola, a world authority on nutrition and biological medicine, has listed them under two headings: the less serious, which are still bothersome, and those which cause serious complications.[10] One can argue with his divisions – depression and increased susceptibility to vaginal and bladder infections when one is dealing with preconception care is hardly 'less serious', but taking both lists together, one can gauge the detrimental effects to female health. His lists include:

'Less serious, although bothersome'
    Increased susceptibility to vaginal and bladder infections.
    Lowered resistance to all infections.
* Cramps.
    Dry, blotchy skin.
    Mouth ulcers.
    Dry, falling hair, and baldness.
    Premature wrinkling.
    Acne.
    Sleep disturbances.
    Inability to concentrate.
* Migraine headaches.
* Depression, moodiness, irritability.

* Darkening of the skin of upper lip and lower eyelids.
* Sore breasts.
* Nausea.
* Weight gain and body distortion due to disproportional distribution of fat.

　Chronic fatigue.
　Increase in dental cavities.
　Swollen and bleeding gums.
* Greatly increased or decreased sex drive.
* Visual disturbances.

　Amenorrhea (no periods).
* Blood sugar level disturbances which complicate diabetes or hypoglycaemia.

'More serious complications'
　Eczema.
　Gallbladder problems.
　Hyperlipemia (excess fat in the blood).
* Intolerance to carbohydrates leading to 'steroid diabetes', which can lead to clinical diabetes.
* Strokes.
* Seven to ten times greater risk of death due to blood clots.
* Jaundice.
* Epilepsy.
* High blood pressure.
* Kidney failure.

　Oedema (swelling).
　Permanent infertility.
* Varicose veins.
* Thrombophlebitis and pulmonary embolism.
* Heart attacks.

　Cancer of the breast, uterus, liver, and pituitary gland.

To this list one can add:
　Vitamin and mineral imbalances.
　Ectopic pregnancy.
　Miscarriage.
　Food allergies.
　Genito-urinary disease, including cervicitis.
　Congenital malformations.
　Osteoporosis.
　Ovarian and lung cancer.[11,12]

You may wonder why some items are asterisked. These are the ones for which there are specific warnings on the instructions which come with all packets of the pill. Obviously, for most women, apart from their doctor, this is where they will get their information about the effects of the pill. It is, therefore, very important that it is not misleading. Yet, if one reads the small print (and it is SMALL PRINT) one can see that the 'facts' are presented very cleverly to minimise the adverse picture painted. For example, in one set of instructions for use,[13] it is claimed that 'Painful periods are in most cases abolished', implying that the user still has periods. Only further down the page is there a phrase which suggests that this is not so, when the 'period' is referred to as a 'period of bleeding resembling a menstrual "period"'. The side effects are referred to as 'occasional', which is certainly not what Grant and others have found. The user is advised to stop taking the pill immediately pregnancy is suspected, because of the risk of congenital abnormality. Does this advice not seem to rest uneasily with the warning earlier in the instructions that 'Not even the combined oral contraceptive can offer 100 per cent protection against pregnancy'. Since we have seen that malformations can arise very early in the pregnancy, stopping after pregnancy will, in many cases, be too late. The text continues: 'It can be definitely concluded, however, that if a risk of abnormality (Fetal malformation) exists at all, it must be very small.' In view of what is known about the effect of hormones on the fetus, this is nonsense. (See below.) The teratogenic effects are underestimated because of the number of miscarriages which occur.

It is impossible, within the constraints of this book, to consider all the above in more detail, so we shall just take some of the more important aspects affecting preconception, conception and the subsequent child. However, you should remember that anything which affects the health of the mother can indirectly, if not directly, affect the health of the fetus.

○ THE PILL AND VITAMIN AND MINERAL IMBALANCES. One of the most widespread deficiencies we have is zinc. (See Chapter 5.) We know it is essential for many biochemical processes in the body, and is especially important in pregnancy. Unfortunately, the pill upsets the balance between copper and zinc levels, raising copper and lowering zinc. Often, therefore, when a woman comes off the pill to become pregnant, she will start at conception in a zinc deficient state, which will get worse as time goes on. This can lead to problems during the gestation for mother and fetus, as well as problems for mother and infant after birth. Difficulties may include post-natal depression and lactation problems in the mother, and feeding difficulties, learning difficulties and developmental difficulties, especially with regard to sexual development for the child. Excess copper has been associated with pre-eclampsia and post-partum depression, among other conditions. The pill also interferes with other minerals, including especially magnesium, also iron, iodine and, probably, chromium and manganese.[14] (See Chapter 5.)

Nor is vitamin metabolism left unscathed. As Grant says: 'Steroids change protein building and breakdown in the liver and change the levels of protein in the blood that carries the vitamins to the body tissues. The pill can alter the actions of the enzymes which need vitamins to function properly.'[15] The pill raises Vitamin A levels, and leads to deficiencies of B1, B2, B3, B6, folic acid and C. It may lower B12.

○ ECTOPIC PREGNANCY. Ectopic pregnancy, a serious condition, which is often life-threatening for the woman, has now reached epidemic-like proportions in the USA[16] and is an increasing worry in the UK. Even where the pregnancy can be successfully aborted, the woman will often have severe Fallopian tube damage or even lose the tube. Some women may have low magnesium levels which may impede tubal muscular action. Some may have infections. There may also be high copper levels.[17]

○ MISCARRIAGE. Pill users have a higher risk of miscarriage even after they have stopped taking the pill, unless specific mineral and vitamin levels are restored to normal. (See Chapter 5.)

○ FOOD ALLERGIES. Although we deal with food allergies in detail in chapter 12, we should emphasise that Grant believes that the pill is a major contributory factor to the increase in food allergy which has now become serious.[18] This is not surprising when one remembers that the pill compromises the immune system leaving it less able to cope with sensitivities. Its effects on liver function mean that enzymes which should help in detoxification do not work properly, thereby exacerbating the effects of toxins from foods and chemicals to which an individual may be allergic. Nutritional imbalances, especially zinc deficiency, are major factors contributing to allergy.

○ GENITO-URINARY INFECTIONS. In Chapter 13, we look in detail at these, including sexually transmitted diseases. Suffice to say here that the pill has led to an increase, not only through greater sexual freedom, but also because of its physical effects on the body. For example, it weakens the immune system so the body is not so resistant to infection. It has, undoubtedly, led to increases in cancers, especially of the cervix in younger than ever women. In part, this is because it was given to many of them when their bodies were still growing, their cervix linings were still immature and susceptible to changes, particularly those leading to cancer.[19]

○ CONGENITAL ABNORMALITIES. Since Dr Isobel Gal first discovered that hormone pregnancy tests, which are no longer used, were associated with higher incidences of congenital malformations of the central nervous system, studies have continued into the teratogenic effects of the pill and other hormones.[20] Some researchers have claimed that recent studies have not confirmed an association,[21,22] although there are others, spanning three continents, which have found statistically significant numbers of abnormalities.

In the USA, researchers found limb-reduction anomalies in one study, with major abnormalities, including congenital heart anomalies and neurological and neural tube disorders in another.[23,24] These findings were confirmed in a major study in Europe, as well as in a number of small ones.[25,26] Other researchers argue that 'Hormonal treatment during pregnancy may be a predisposing factor in congenital heart defects'.[29] Even researchers of studies which failed to find links warn that there is a need for further studies.[30,31]

○ FERTILITY. The pill interferes with the hormone system to prevent pregnancy. However, even after a woman has ceased taking it, the body's systems may not return to normal. Having had the message to switch off making certain hormones for so long, the body takes time to adjust to producing them again. Sadly for some women, the adjustment may take a long time, or may never happen. Nutritional imbalances, especially zinc deficiency, are also often a factor. (See Chapter 15.)

Intra-uterine devices – the IUD, or coil

The IUD is a small device, which is inserted into the womb by a doctor. There are many shapes in use, made from more or less toxic materials such as plastic, copper, or plastic-coated copper. Its continual presence in the womb prevents conception, though it is still not clear how. It may prevent the egg from attaching to the lining of the womb by mechanical means, or it may be by some toxic action. Its failure rate is higher than the pill. It is also quite harmful, the side effects including:

- Cramping and pain, especially during menstruation.
- Ectopic pregnancy (pregnancy occurring outside the womb).
- Spontaneous abortion.
- Uterine bleeding.
- Blood poisoning.
- Bowel obstruction.
- Cervical infection (and infection of the uterus).
- Pelvic infections.
- Infections in the Fallopian tubes.
- Dysplasia.
- Cancer of the uterus.
- Anaemia.
- Perforation of the uterus.
- It can become imbedded in the uterus, which often means hospitalisation and even death.
- Mineral imbalances, especially elevated copper and low zinc.[32]

In an attempt to overcome some of these problems, sometimes chemicals, such as progesterone or progestogen, are added. As the section on the pill has shown, though, this is not a safe practice. Many of the side effects are caused or exacerbated by poor fitting. Users may also find it difficult to check its position.

Clearly, when it comes to preconception care and pregnancy, many of the above are undesirable. The problems associated with infections are discussed elsewhere (see Chapter 13), as are the problems of excess copper and zinc deficiency (see Chapter 5).

Conclusion
No contraceptive method which interferes with the chemistry and physiology of the body, as do the pill and the IUD, can be recommended. It is impossible to calculate how much iatrogenic illness (illness caused by medical intervention) is caused by them, especially the pill. The evidence for the harm they do is overwhelming and well documented in the medical literature. You should not be fooled by anyone who tells you otherwise! Remember that a number of countries will not permit their use.

Checklist
1. If you have never taken the pill, don't be persuaded to start.
2. If you have taken the pill in the past, it is advisable, regardless of whether or not you are pregnant, that you have a check-up with a doctor who is trained to recognise mineral imbalances. If you are breastfeeding it is especially important.
3. Until your body is in balance, it would be preferable for you to avoid pregnancy, but by methods other than the pill. (See Chapter 6.)

CHAPTER 10

Physical and Chemical Hazards in the Workplace and Home

INFORMATION YOU NEED TO CHECK OUT AT WORK AND AT HOME — IS IT SAFE FOR THE UNBORN BABY?

Some years ago if you opened a book on occupational health you would rarely find a mention of reproductive hazards. Now, with women of child-bearing age forming a large part of the workforce, and with recognition that occupational hazards can affect the male reproductive system, there are whole books on the subject, as well as large parts of others. The hazards are many, ranging from physical ones, such as radiation, VDUs, noise, light and heat, to chemical ones, such as formaldehyde and benzene. Some are associated with particular occupations. The home is also not without its dangers, some brought in from the workplace, others from the environment, including in the shopping bag.

There are, however, two key points that can be made generally. Firstly, prenatal exposure is more likely to produce toxic effects than adult exposure, so that the pregnant woman may not seem to have health problems herself, although her child may be affected. Secondly, as we saw in the chapter on toxic metals (see Chapter 7), exposure to chemicals in the workplace can cause behavioural changes even without any physical signs of damage. One authority has suggested that 'detection of behavioural deviations in children of mothers exposed to a hazardous substance while pregnant may be one of the most sensitive indicators of toxicity'.[1] In this chapter we focus on the main hazards. There is considerable overlap with subjects covered elsewhere in the text. Lead, for example, is a major industrial toxin, used in many processes. Many of the industrial pollutants can cause allergic reactions which undermine the immune system and general health. But before turning to the chemical hazards, we consider the physical factors, including radiation, which generates so much fear.

Ionising radiation

Rays of ionising radiation include alpha, beta and gamma rays, neutrons and X-rays. They are so powerful that they shatter atoms they touch, causing them to lose electrons, thereby developing an electric charge. These charged particles are called ions, hence the term 'ionising'. Because of their power they are extremely damaging to tissues in the body, and can cause death quickly or slowly. They penetrate the body without a person knowing. They hit atoms and molecules, breaking them up to form free radicals and oxidising agents. These two chemical groups may be quite damaging as they break up proteins, destroy chromosomes and change other chemicals. The results may be death of the cells, immediately or earlier than the usual lifespan, changes in the growth and division of the cell such that there may be no growth or uncontrolled growth (cancer), or prominent changes in the way the cell works.

Man has always been exposed to some ionising radiation. However, Dr Rosalie Bertell has pointed out that the 'natural' levels have increased from an exposure of 60 millirem a year in 1940 to 100 in the 1950s to 200 millirems in the 1980s – mainly due to weapons testing.[2] Not all scientists agree with her figures, but no one disputes that more of us are exposed to more radiation than ever before, if only because of the increased use of X-rays and nuclear medicine. There is also a large amount of low level radiation in many industries that may have seemed innocuous. Indeed, some 6,000 sites are approved as being able to handle radioactive materials in the UK, including schools and factories. Sometimes workers are not told they are handling radioactive materials: in some areas, materials are dumped without proper authority and protection for nearby residents.[3]

Frequently we are reassured that low doses, such as that received in an X-ray, are safe. But the truth is that *no* level of radiation has been proved safe, and it is likely that *any* level is potentially harmful. Dr Bertell worries that scientists only ask about the risks of cancer from radiation exposure when it has other, more serious effects. She is especially concerned about the genetic pool:

'Children are now being born weakened by radioactivity, prone to enzyme disorders, allergies and asthma directly caused by cell mutations.' She talks of a weakened new generation less able to cope with an ever increasing dose of radiation in the environment. 'By the fifth generation of children born into the post-nuclear age the damage to the entire gene pool will be very clear indeed.'

She denounces the international 'safety' level that power stations work to: '...maximum 500 millirems a year to the public or plant workers...equivalent to 100 chest X-rays'.[4] Other researchers have also indicated that even increases in background radioactivity, within natural levels, may have damaging effects on the fetus and may be a reason for higher malformation rates.[5]

X-rays have been the subject of much research and concern, especially since Dr Alice Stewart shows that they could harm the fetus, causing a high risk of childhood leukemia.[6] Animal research confirms these adverse effects, in both males and females. When mature eggs of female mice were irradiated the offspring had a high incidence of cancer.[7] Where dominant mutations have been produced in male germ cells by X-rays, low birth weight results.[8]

Non-ionising radiation

Non-ionising rays, including ultra violet, infra red, lasers, microwaves, radar, radio frequency waves and extra low frequency waves, are produced naturally by the sun and also created in the home, in industry and in military use. Although not powerful enough to create ions, no one should be fooled about their safety. The chief of research of non-ionising radiation at the National Institute of Environmental Health Sciences, North Carolina, Donald McRee, has said:

> In animal experiments, (the Russians) have found that this radiation causes changes in almost every system: behaviour, blood chemistry, the endocrine functions, reproductive organs, and the immune system. In studies of human workers exposed to microwave equipment for many years, they have reported abnormally slow heart beats, chest pains, and birth defects. And they've found a lot of more subjective effects, things like insomnia, irritability, headaches, and loss of memory.[9]

Of major concern to us here are sunlight, ultra violet, microwaves, radar and radio frequency waves.

Sunlight

'Light is a primal element of life.'[10] Indeed, without it we would not have life as we know it. We tend to talk about the benefits of 'fresh air' without being aware of the beneficial effects of natural light. Yet research has shown that natural light and artificial light have different physiological effects in animals, including human beings, which show in a variety of physical and mental conditions, such as tumours and hyperactivity.

Clearly, artificial lighting is an essential part of modern lifestyles. But it is possible to buy full-spectrum lighting, which is very similar to natural light and quite different from fluorescent, neon and other artificial forms. (See Appendix One for addresses.) Full-spectrum lighting covers more specific wavelengths, especially the blue or ultra violet ones that are missing from artificial lighting. (See below.) If they are blocked out, an endocrine deficiency can arise.[11] Mice kept in artificial light conditions died prematurely or had very small litters, suggesting the need for further research.[12] Full-spectrum lighting has been shown to help alleviate seasonal affective depression.[13] It has also been used in a classroom to reduce hyperactivity.[14] Sunlight has been found to help with the elimination of toxic metals from the body, and the metabolism of desirable minerals.[15]

Ultra violet

Ultra violet rays can be UV-A or UV-B type. The UV-B are the ones that give you sunburn, but although UV-A is weaker, one expert says it does the same damage, and may even be worse. To get brown, you need the same overall exposure, so with UV-A, it just means that you will have to sunbathe longer. However, UV-A penetrates deeper than UV-B, and may cause damage to collagen, blood vessels and elastic tissues. UV-B may therefore be safer, because the UV-A lulls you into a false sense of security. Also, once exposed to UV-A, the body is more susceptible to the aging and carcinogenic effects of UV-B radiation.[16]

There is now quite a scare about sunbathing and skin cancer. To induce skin cancer in animals, it is necessary to give larger-than-normal doses of ultra violet light so that burning occurs.[17] There also seems to be a direct relationship between the amount of free radicals formed in the skin when it is exposed to sunlight and the tendency for that skin to burn. Stop the free radicals forming and you considerably reduce the sunburning. Another factor that may be significant is cholesterol, which may be changed into a number of products when the ultra violet strikes the skin, one of which, cholesterol alphaoxide, can act as a free radical and cause cancer.[18] (Free radical formation can be inhibited by certain nutrients in the diet, such as Vitamins A, C and E.) Oils and fats applied to the skin, or sunbathing creams may also stimulate cancer formation.[19]

So should you avoid ultra violet light? This is not the good idea that the advertisements would have us believe, since it means avoiding natural sunlight, or at least parts of it, and the ultra violet portion is the most biologically active. Ultra violet wavelengths can kill bacteria, and infections are definitely to be avoided in pregnancy![20] Ultra violet treatments are provided by law to miners in Russia, as they have been found to help remove dust from the lungs.[21]

Visual display units – VDUs

VDUs are widely used in the workplace and home. There is considerable debate over their safety, especially for the pregnant woman, but few conclusions can be drawn. Studies have produced mixed results, though one reason may be that the testing is not always done on machines as they are used – perhaps neglected, unserviced and without proper safety precautions. They may release low levels of radiation, including X-rays, microwaves, ultra violet and infra red light.[22] Although some authorities argue that these levels are too low to cause harm, Mr Tony Webb, a noted expert on the subject, disagrees: 'There is no safe level of radiation. In addition, there is no conclusive evidence that these low levels do not cause damage.'[23]

Worries about birth defects and VDUs arose from reports of an apparently high number of birth defects among a group of VDU operators in Canada in 1980. Other studies have revealed clusters, including one among staff at the Department of Employment in Cheshire, where in 55 pregnancies in VDU users, 14.5 per cent ended with a miscarriage, 6.7 per cent in stillbirth and 22 per cent in some kind of malformation. For women not using VDUs the figures were 5.3 per cent less than 1 per cent and 11 per cent respectively.[24] However, there were reservations about the statistics. It may be that VDU operators suffer high levels of stress, especially if they work uninterrupted for long periods. Stress is known to be a risk factor in pregnancy. In other countries, notably Scandinavia and the USA, employers are seeking ways of limiting their employees' exposure to VDU radiation.[25] This can be done by regular rest periods, protective equipment to reduce the rays emitted, and shielding of the operator with special clothing. It would seem sensible if these precautions were standard procedure, since with what we know about low level radiation, we are unlikely to prove conclusively that VDUs are not potentially harmful.

Microwaves (see also Chapter 11)
Microwaves are energy waves that are used in many different types of equipment, especially in telecommunications, e.g. radar. Microwaves can penetrate deeply into the body, causing its temperature to rise. High intensity microwaves can lead to permanent damage. For example, the heat generated can cause the cell lining of the testicles to degenerate, thereby damaging them.[26] It is also suspected of causing breast cancer, especially where a microwave oven is placed at breast height.[27] The problem arises because the breast (and eyes) have a poor blood supply so the heat is not dissipated. Microwaves may also cause genetic damage: one study has shown that more Down's syndrome children were fathered by men exposed to microwaves than to fathers not so exposed.[28] (See also Chapter 11.)

Electricity
People living near high-voltage power lines have sometimes complained that their health was affected by them, though this has been dismissed as nonsense! However, in March 1988, the Chairman of the Central Electricity Generating Board launched a £500,000 study into the effects of high-voltage lines on health. At the launch, though, officials were still being dismissive of the likelihood of any link, though other countries accept the risks that the electromagnetic fields generated by them can damage health.[29] Russia limits the time a farm worker can spend near them to three hours, while the USA will not allow houses to be built near them.[30] One group of researchers found an increase in all birth defects for conceptions that occurred during the time the father worked on high-voltage systems.[31] Another suggested an association between the use of electric blankets and infertility and birth defects. They hypothesised that strong electromagnetic fields may be generated by electric blankets under certain circumstances. The seasonal variation of rates of births and birth defects may agree with the time periods of peak electric blanket use.[32] (Of course, they may also peak with many other factors, such as reduced sunlight or different food availability.)

Heat

Extremes of heat and cold cause stress to the body, which can be disadvantageous in preconception care. But as well as these general stress effects, there may be specific ones associated with heat.

In the man, heat can interfere with sperm production, since the testicles need to operate at a lower temperature than the rest of the body. Hours of sitting, such as happens with taxi and lorry drivers, travelling salesmen and business executives, may result in excess scrotal heat.[33] Skin-tight underwear or frequent hot baths can have a similar effect.[34]

In the woman, a high body temperature (hyperthermia) can cause damage to the fetus. Hyperthermia tends to stop the division of cells and very high temperatures may even kill cells.[35] In the fetus, cell division is basic to growth, so stopping it can have devastating consequences. Both brain size and function have been affected.

High temperatures may occur with infections and people have queried if problems arise as a result of the infection or the high temperature itself. Research suggests the latter alone can cause damage. One study of brain damaged children revealed that their healthy mothers had taken regular prolonged saunas. The researchers suggest that prolonged saunas should be avoided during the first three to five months of pregnancy.[36] Short saunas, six to ten minutes long, such as are taken by the Finns, seem safe.

Noise

A Japanese study of 1,000 births linked lower birth weights with noise and lower levels of certain hormones believed to affect the fetal growth.[37] It is not known what levels of maternal noise exposure may harm the fetus. Certainly, since 1935, it has been known that the effects of sound in general affect the fetus, when it was shown that a doorbell buzzer applied to the woman's abdomen in the last two months of pregnancy resulted in hyperactivity for the fetus and an increased fetal heart rate.[38]

We do need, however, to put noise in context – noise levels in these settings was loud enough to cause undue stress to the body. The fetus is not growing in a noise-free environment: it is subjected to the noises in its mother's body, as well as those from her normal day-to-day activities.[39] Some cultures, and many mothers, believe that soft soothing sounds are beneficial to the baby's development. Noise at general levels is part of your baby's stimulation!

Chemical hazards

A guiding principle when considering the matter of chemical hazards in reproduction must be the point made by Dr Joan Spyker, an eminent toxicologist: 'Nearly every chemical to which the pregnant woman is exposed will ultimately reach the fetus.'[40] We must also remember that the fetus does not have a mature system to detoxify all the poisons that may be passed to it.

Some of the hazards are discussed elsewhere in this book – lead, cadmium, drugs and organophosphates, for example. Here we focus on others known or suspected of causing harm in reproduction. It is not easy to do good studies, and many of the long-term effects are not known. Even where they are it can be difficult to eradicate the offending substance – organochlorides, pesticides, are a pertinent example. (See Chapter 11.) We may have banned the use of DDT in Britain and the USA but we still manufacture and export it to the Third World only to import the food on which it has been used.*

Let us look closer at some of the more hazardous substances.

a. *Chlorinated pesticides,* such as Kepone and DBCP. These have been found to produce low sperm counts, defective sperm and sterility.[42,43] Fortunately, those workers exposed to Kepone eventually recovered: sadly, those exposed to DBCP often suffered irreversible testicular damage.[44] Although DBCP and DDT are banned in Britain we still permit the use of Lindane, known to cause fetal cancer.[45] Since they are regularly found in food samples, it is possible for sperm counts to be lowered simply by eating food from your regular sources. (See Chapter 11.)

b. *Polychlorinated biphenyls (PCBs).* Now banned in Britain, these were widely used in industry because of their specific properties, one of which was their resistance to biodegradation. This has, unfortunately, made them ubiquitous. These have been found in high quantities in semen samples and are now linked with low sperm counts, poor fetal growth, low birth weight, or poor survival rates.[46] like the organochlorides, they are fat-soluble so can be found in high concentrations in breast milk.[47] The advice offered to mothers who are worried about breastfeeding is to carry on, but not to try to lose weight while doing so, to avoid mobilising too much fat. The fact is that substitute milks are also contaminated, but they do not offer the other protective substances that human milk contains.

The disposal of PCBs is now a problem. Although burning is the best way, it releases small quantities of dioxin, which is even more dangerous to health. Dumping at sea is not a solution, because they find their way into fatty fish.

c. *Vinyl chloride.* Widely used in more than half of all plastic products, these should not be confused with polyvinyl chloride, which has not yet been found hazardous, except to people with chemical sensitivities. Vinyl chlorides are linked with loss of libido in workers, and a higher than usual incidence of neural tube defects has been reported in some towns with factories producing them, possibly reflecting damage to the sperm.[48] There are also high numbers of fetal deaths, and wives have a high rate of miscarriage. Decreased libido, impotence, decreased fetal growth, low birth weight and poor survival rates have been mentioned.[49] They are known animal teratogens.[50]

---

*Concern about pesticides led Sir Richard Body, former chairman of the House of Commons Select Committee on Agriculture, to submit (with others) a report on the subject.[41]

d. *Chloroprene*. These have been linked with decreased libido, impotence, testicular damage, and infertility in the man and menstrual and other gynaecological disorders in the woman.[51]

e. *Formaldehyde*. These are associated with menstrual and other gynaecological problems, abortions, infertility, decreased fetal growth, low birth weight or poor survival.[52]

f. *Solvents*. Solvents include the aromatic hydrocarbons such as benzene and tuolene. Many working women receive a double dose – at work and in the home. Some are linked with decreased libido and impotence in the man, while in the woman some can cause menstrual and other gynaecological problems, with benzene being linked to maternal deaths related to pregnancy.[53] Benzene can damage the chromosomes and is possibly teratogenic.[54] They may also be a factor in decreased fetal growth, low birth weight and poor survival rates.[55] Solvents were the presumed hazard in a study from Sweden, which reported that women in medical laboratories had more risk of spontaneous abortion and, perhaps, birth defects. They may also have been responsible for some spontaneous abortions among New York cleaners, although the stress of physical work could have been a factor too.[56] (See below.)

g. *Dimethylformamide* – DMF. This chemical is used in the production of paint, artificial fibres, drugs, and as a solvent in leather dyes, pesticides and many other products. It is linked with testicular cancer.[57]

Of course, many of these chemicals are found in the home in food, in the form of additives (see Chapter 11), in cleaning products, in materials used for DIY and hobbies and in the garden. We may request food free from additives, then spray insecticides over our own gardens and in our homes in the form of flysprays! We may complain about the way industry pollutes the planet, but then we use a spray polish, which releases solvents into the atmosphere! We may complain about lead in the atmosphere, and then ignore the lead-free pump at the petrol station!

It may not be possible to eliminate all such substances from the home, but it is possible to limit their use. They are not as essential as we have come to believe, though some of the alternatives may not be as quick to use. They will, however, be much cheaper, as well as being kinder to the planet! Friends of the Earth and Greenpeace are only two of the organisations which can offer advice. (See Appendix One for addresses.) It is possible to buy alternatives, such as Ecover products, or you can make your own. We give below a few suggestions mostly taken from a Greenpeace leaflet[58]:

Cleaners: All purpose cleaner – 1 gallon hot water with 50 ml each of ammonia and vinegar, and 15 ml baking soda. Never mix with other cleaners. Use gloves.

Laundry: Use soap and/or washing soda.

Polish: Dissolve 1 teaspoon of lemon oil in a pint of mineral oil.
  Use sparingly with a clean rag.
  Use a cloth wetted with vinegar.

Dishes: Use soap flakes in hot water, adding vinegar for heavy grease.
Garden pests: Handpicking is best. You can also consult the organic gardening guides by the Henry Doubleday Research centre. (See Appendix One.) (Because of government regulations, we cannot tell you of the many traditional ways, since the government argues that they have not been subjected to proper testing for toxicity!)

Specific occupational risks

An Office of Population and Censuses Surveys (OPCS) report looked at the abnormal reproductive aspects of a large number of occupations, some of which were already known but are often overlooked. Both male and female chemical and gas petroleum process plant operators had raised incidences of congenital malformations in their offspring. Road transport drivers had raised risks of Down's syndrome, CNS malformations, clefts and cardiovascular conditions. Welders were shown to have a high incidence of spina bifida children (though not other malformations), sudden infant death and abnormal sex ratio. Textile workers have fairly high rates of stillbirth and perinatal infant mortality. Publicans have raised risks of cleft malformations, possibly due to the alcohol (though they are generally in smoky atmospheres too).[59] The list could go on ...

Often overlooked are the hazards in offices – the gases emitted by photocopiers, the outgassing of carbonated paper, not to mention all the symptoms associated with 'Sick Building Syndrome'.[60,61] Then there are the potential physical hazards of poor lighting, bad seating, VDU strain, noise and overcrowding.

But if office hazards have been generally ignored, this is not the case in operating theatres, which have been the subject of much research. Even so, there are disagreements about the reproductive dangers, with some contradictory results. However, a survey by the American Society of Anesthesiologists found that nurses working in operating theatres had a 60 per cent higher rate of deformed children compared with nurses in other departments, while female anaesthetists had twice as many deformed children as other female physicians. 25 per cent more male anaesthetists had deformed children compared with other physicians.[62] Female dental surgeons have also been found to have high rates of miscarriage, probably as a result of exposure to anaesthetics, though dentists are generally at risk from mercury toxicity. (See Chapter 7.) Fortunately, it is possible to modify machines to reduce toxic emissions.

Airline pilots are often at risk of temporary infertility which a period of grounding can remove.

Specific hazardous environments

Many of these will be obvious! If you live near a chemical factory you probably know you do. It may well not be possible for you to move, but you may be able to reduce the hazards by local actions, such as through your environmental health officer's monitoring, as well as your own. It is known that some specific locations do seem to have extra risks associated with them.

Airports
Excessive numbers of stillbirths were reported around Heathrow Airport, while near Osaka airport, Japan, there were high numbers of low weight babies. The idea that airports have adverse prenatal effects was supported by a large study done in the Los Angeles area in 1978, which showed that the rate of birth defects in the vicinity of the airport was almost 12 per thousand births, as opposed to a rate of seven per thousand births for the remainder of the Los Angeles county.[63]

Military installations
Fort Rucker is a military aviation centre where a high number of defects were found in children of helicopter pilots. They are exposed to many more microwaves than ground staff, as they fly low. There were also other defects in children of military staff based there.[64]

There are still arguments about why these environments should be more hazardous. One expert believes that the Los Angeles figures are the result of high noise levels, while another thinks it is due to the microwaves which abound where there is radar.[65] At Fort Rucker, there are 48 radar installations within a 30-mile radius. The truth probably lies in a combination of a number of factors.

Farms
We tend to think of the countryside as healthier than the town, and this is probably true. But if you are living next to an intensively run farm you should be wary of agrochemicals. Check with the farmer on the sprays, etc, he uses. Ask to be informed when he is using them. Make sure he and his staff know their dangers.

Nuclear power stations, and factories which emit fumes and gases
These have been the subject of much argument, especially with regard to childhood cancers. There is still no conclusive proof that they are harmful. *But neither is there any proof that they are harmless.* Indeed, no adequate explanations have been offered for the clusters of disease that sometimes occur. Maybe you should think twice about moving to an area that could be affected if you have a choice.

Checklist
With all the many hazards in our everyday lives, it is important to recognise that we must keep a balance. We cannot avoid all of them, so we must take sensible precautions, without being over-worried.
1. Know what products you work with, what their dangers are and obey all safety regulations. If you are concerned, speak to your

employer, trade union official or environmental health officer.
2. Look for alternative safe products to use.
3. Always use products in accordance with the manufacturer's instructions – if it says 'Do not use in confined spaces', DON'T.
4. Keep all toxins locked away in their original containers.

CHAPTER 11

Food Production

HELP IN RECOGNISING THE HAZARDS — HOW TO AVOID THEM — WHY TO AVOID THEM — WHAT TO DO NEXT.

Chapter 5 stressed the importance of wholesome food in maintaining health, especially that of the fetus. It emphasised the need for food to be grown on healthy soil, and eaten as close to its natural state as possible. In this chapter we support our belief in these principles by explaining how food is produced – from the seed to the table.

Soil

Lady Eve Balfour, former president of the Soil Association, highlighted what others had said for many years – *the soil is a living organism*. Like our three pioneers (see Chapter 5), she said that 'the health of man, beast, plant and soil is one indivisible whole; that the health of the soil depends on maintaining its biological balance'.[1] Over-reliance on agrochemicals does not treat our soil as a living organism. These substances kill the organisms which live in the soil breaking down the decaying matter into nutrients for the plants, and they create imbalances which eventually erode the soil. This leads to a vicious circle, since farmers counteract lower productivity by more agrochemicals, further exhausting the soil. The agrochemicals unbalance the mineral structure, since the over-cropping encouraged by them reduces the levels of some trace elements, as well as raising the levels of nitrogen, potassium and phosphorus. They do nothing to add to the organic content of the soil, which reduces its water-retaining capacity, thereby rendering it more vulnerable to erosion. Eventually it can take no more and becomes barren.[2] Other techniques which are the result of an agrochemical approach, such as the uprooting of hedges for easier access by larger machinery, contribute to soil erosion. It is true to say that there are large barren areas where there was once fertility. It is possible to regain fertility but this takes time and money. The Soil Association reckons on an average of five years to convert a farm to organic methods, though it could be two years if there has been little damage to the soil structure or longer if there has been extensive damage.

Of course, trace element problems arise from a number of environmental sources. There are the natural occurrences, such as low iodine in Derbyshire, which caused many cases of goitre (Derbyshire neck) until the reason became known. Industrial processes, including mining and smelter waste, can build up toxins. (See Chapter 7.) Pulverised fuel ash may lead to high levels of arsenic, boron, aluminium and copper, which can be toxic to young plants. Pesticides, fungicides and other agrochemicals can build up high levels of mercury, lead and arsenic. Sewerage sludge may be contaminated with toxic metals. Animal wastes, from animals who are not reared organically, may result in imbalances: zinc and copper levels may be raised, because of their use in pig and poultry feeds. (But see below.)[3] There is now a great deal of concern over the amounts and effects of nitrates and nitrites. Nitrates are known 'to alter and stabilise the chemical structure of haemoglobin, so that it is unable to bind and release oxygen'. There is also concern that they may cause stomach cancer.[4] In general, the six most important trace elements needed by field crops are iron, manganese, boron, zinc, copper and molybdenum. The availability to the plant of both zinc and iron can be affected by high levels of soil phosphorus.[5] Thus, since agrochemicals contain only nitrogen, potassium and phosphorus, the other trace elements, which should be available to us in the plants we eat, are lost by two routes – firstly, through the unbalanced fertilisers which do not replace the trace elements lost and, secondly, through the action of the unbalanced fertilisers on the bioavailability of the trace elements. Zinc, for example, so important in health and reproduction, has become quite deficient in many soils because of a failure to maintain the organic structure of the soil and the use of agrochemicals.[6] Liming reduces the level of manganese in leafy vegetables.[7]

There are many studies which show that foods produced by ecological methods contain more nutrients than those grown by agrochemical methods.[8] The Soil Association can give details of them, as well as provide lists of sources of organic foods.

Seed

Seeds are subject to many regulations, including patenting. EEC membership has restricted the number of varieties which are allowed to be grown, though you can legally grow lost varieties for research. It is no exaggeration to say that hundreds, if not thousands, of plants have been lost to the British market, with serious consequences. With the growth of large-scale agriculture, plant breeders are more concerned with plants which will have a uniform colour, all ripen together, are easily harvested using modern machinery, are easily stored and travel well. (The ultimate must be the square tomato developed in California!) This has led to plants which require considerable agrochemical input, with all its dangers. Old varieties of seed survived because they had been selected for specific qualities, having shown they could adapt to a certain set of circumstances. If their genes are lost, the ability to benefit from these qualities in later varieties is lost also – qualities which may be essential in the future, given the changes in climate, soil and techniques.[9] Some varieties thrive in wet climates, others in dry. Some need a long growing season, others a short. There is nothing wrong with trying to combine varieties to get the best from each – farmers have selected their best seed each year for centuries. However, it is widely agreed that an agrochemical agricultural system cannot be sustained in the long term, so it is shortsighted to breed only varieties dependent on such chemicals. Seed patenting and EEC restrictive regulations are not ensuring a broad gene pool for the future.

This situation has arisen because most seed companies are now owned by the large oil companies who make the agrochemicals. Such restrictive practices are in their interests alone. Unfortunately they have power to pressure the EEC to impose further restrictions and they have shown that they are unscrupulous enough to use it.[10,11]

The growing plant

Drawing on the nutrients in a healthy soil, and given the right moisture and appropriate climate, the seed should develop into a plant healthy enough to resist attacks from diseases and predators. Where organic methods are being introduced, it may be necessary to have some form of pest control, but there are products which do not harm the environment or which are selective in the insects they kill. (See Appendix Two for recommended reading.)

There are a number of good reasons for farming and gardening without the use of agrochemicals (some of which have been discussed above but which are worth repeating):

- They harm the environment, indiscriminately killing organisms in the soil. Insects, birds, animals and human beings are also harmed.
- They destroy the soil structure.
- They adversely affect human health since the body is exposed to a multiplicity of new chemicals in amounts never before encountered by whole populations, and for which the body's detoxification systems were not designed.
- They are expensive.

Unfortunately, though, most of the produce we eat has been exposed to some sort of agrochemical – grown with artificial fertilisers and treated with pesticides, such as herbicides, fungicides and insecticides, based often on organophosphates. Just how damaging are these pesticides? We answer that by looking more closely at insecticides, though fungicides, which often contain mercury (see Chapter 7), and herbicides are also based on organophosphorus.[12]

Pesticides

Organochlorides, such as DDT, were hailed as the saviour of the farmers, in their drive to meet ever-increasing demands for better quality cheap food. However, as their detrimental effects were realised, especially following the publication of Rachel Carson's classic *Silent Spring*, their use became restricted or banned, leading to an increased use of organophosphorous pesticides (organophosphates). (But remember that the manufacturers have no qualms about selling those chemicals banned in the UK or USA to Third World countries!)

The insecticide properties of organophosphates were discovered in 1937, although the chemicals on which they are based had originally been developed by the Germans in the First World War as potential nerve gas. Since the 1960s, formulae less toxic to man have been developed for use in pest control. But we should not be fooled into equating 'less toxic' with 'non-toxic'. The truth is that organophosphates cause great harm to human beings.

They work by inactivating various enzyme systems in the organisms which ingest them.[13] But they cannot discriminate between organisms so man is affected by them as well as the insects at which their poisonous effects are directed.

The main enzymes affected are:

1. Cholinesterase, which is responsible for hydrolysing acetylcholine from choline. It is interesting to note that cholinesterase is found in high concentrations in the spinal cord of fetal lambs and humans during the development of the spinal cord. It only increases in the brain-stem and brain shortly before birth.[14] (See Chapter 5.)
2. Liver enzymes. The synergistic effects of two organophosphates can be especially damaging, as can the situation where a drug is given which has toxic side effects for the liver.
3. Neurotoxic esterase (NTE). This enzyme activity is not only inhibited, but there will also be changes in the structure and function of the affected nerves.[15]

Obviously, substances which affect such a wide range of enzymes will result in a large variety of conditions. in studies of animals and humans who have been intentionally or accidentally exposed, many effects have been reported, including ataxia, brain dysfunction, irreversible delayed neurotoxicity, damage to the nerve axon, increased secretion from the nasolacrimal glands, bronchial glands, sweat glands, gastrointestinal glands, bronchoconstriction, cardiovascular problems, such as hypotension, skeletal problems, restlessness, tremor, tonic/clonic convulsions, abnormal reflexes, respiratory and cardiac depression, coma, emotional lability, visual hallucinations, increased libido, excessive dreaming, peripheral weakness, lesions of the myelin sheath (suggesting a role in multiple sclerosis perhaps), memory loss, depression, schizophrenic reactions and inappropriate focusing of attention, long-term change in brain function and death.[16-19] The list is not exhaustive, but it is horrifying enough! If one adds the reactions found in cattle which have been treated with organophosphorus warble fly dressings one can add: paralysis – incoordination, skin lesions, depressed milk yield, bloat, abdominal distress, excessive salivation, no remastication, anorexia, hypermotility of the intestines and diarrhoea, rapid breathing, muscle twitching, shivering, stilted movement, weakness, ataxia of the hind legs with tail head raised, but the rest limp, periods of excitement and depression, bradycardia and urination. In more severe cases, the animal tends to fall around with paddling of the legs: inactivation of the body and limbs follows, with the head and neck being swung from side to side. The side effects may last for several days. One researcher has said that the incidence rate was one per 46,000 animals.[20] However, one farmer argues that the incidence is much higher.[21] (Not all animals will be afflicted in the same way as they are all biochemically different – see Chapter 5.)

There are regulations laid down about the use of these chemicals, but they are hardly realistic. When did you last see a notice near fields suggesting that you did not walk past without protective clothing, while spraying was going on? A market garden known to one of the authors (SGB) displayed a notice on its greenhouse warning people not to stray from the public footpath which ran beside it because it had been sprayed with a chemical containing methyl-mercury. But it did not seem to consider the problem of drift. In March 1988, the Ministry of Agriculture, Fisheries and Food banned the sale of weedkillers containing ioxynil and bromoxynil, two chemicals suspected of being teratogens. But it was not a total ban, only applying to garden weedkillers. Farmers and their workers were still allowed to use it, though they were not permitted to apply it with hand-held sprayers. It was reported that 'labels on professionally-used pesticide products containing the chemicals are to be altered to reduce the risk of residues in food and to warn users of possible fish poisoning'.[22] Should we be reassured? We do not have access to figures on residue levels: they are secret. But the Association of Public Analysts, which conducts tests for the Ministry, found residues in one-third of the fresh fruit and vegetables it tested in 1983, and the level was regarded as significant in a seventh of all the samples collected.[23] More recent checks have been equally disturbing.[24] (See also Chapter 12.)

Harvesting the crop
Assuming that all has gone well with the plants, they will be harvested. One could be naïve and expect this to happen when they are ripe. But that will not necessarily bring in the greatest return for the food industry. It is on this point that the harvesting depends! Thus crops are often picked before they are ripe, to be ripened off later by one or more of the various physical or chemical treatments. Such treatments can also be used to delay ripening.[25] The crop may also be damaged by machinery during harvesting.

Storing the crop
Ideally grains should be sun-dried after harvesting. Florence Nightingale always insisted that 'wheat, barley, oats, maize and millet purchased for the Army in India must be freshly harvested, be clean

and have a moisture content of under 10 per cent'.[26] If grains are not dried off properly, moulds may develop, which may produce harmful substances called mycotoxins. These can cross the placenta and may induce abnormalities in the fetus, depending on how advanced the pregnancy is. Some act like oestrogens and have long-term effects like the pill. (See Chapter 9.) Others are irritants, causing indigestion, swelling of the mouth and digestive tract, with bleeding. Some mycotoxins are produced in high humidity and in temperatures which are found in this country's intervention stores. (See below.) They can form in refrigerated temperatures above 5 degrees centigrade. Some are not destroyed in cooking and scraping the mouldy layer off food is no protection, as they can penetrate the food below.[27]

Since we grow vast surpluses of cereals, the best of the surplus goes into intervention or storage. In order to keep it for long periods, it will often be sprayed with fungicides. These can be as injurious to health as the moulds they are destroying. Fruit and vegetables are also sprayed to enable them to be stored for longer periods and to eliminate rotting before sale.[28] Insecticides may also be used to prevent destruction by pests.[29]

Immediately after harvest the crop may be subjected to precooling or the rapid removal of field heat to slow deterioration possibly by rapidly moving air, ice, cooling by water or vacuum. The food has now become a 'product'[30] which may now undergo processing.

Prolonged storage, even in optimum conditions, reduces the nutritional value of the food. Lettuces stored in a refrigerator lose 50 per cent of their Vitamin C in three days. Asparagus, broccoli and green beans lose 50 per cent of their Vitamin C before reaching the greengrocer.[31]

Before we turn to processing methods, let us backtrack to the farm again, this time to animal production, which follows many similar practices.

Animal production

Just as grains and vegetables are different from those of our grandparents, so meat and poultry have changed and become dependent on chemicals. Intensive farming means that we eat inferior meat and poultry because we are eating unhealthy animals. They are reared on drugs to stimulate quick growth, and kept in overcrowded conditions to increase numbers, which means they are prone to disease. To forestall this, the farmer uses antibiotics on a regular basis, supposedly as a preventive measure. But this prevention may mean that the antibiotic may not work as a cure when we have a disease, as we have been consuming so much of the antibiotic in our food that it ceases to have any effect when needed for medicinal purposes. Chloramphenicol is used to treat scours, a virulent salmonella infection in cattle. It is banned in animal feed in the USA because it is the only treatment known for typhoid in man. It is also known to cause fatal aplastic anaemia and/or leukemia in man. It is not banned in the UK.[32]

Antibiotics in poultry actually promote growth, so are added to feedstuff as a matter of course.[33]

Hormones have proved especially hazardous for the unborn child. The first synthetic hormone, stilbenes (DES), was found to cause cancer in children after their mothers had been given it during pregnancy. When it was later used in animals, babies and young children had abnormal sexual development.[34] Yet more hormones were developed, though they are banned in many European countries because their effects are not understood. Britain, Canada, the USA, France and Ireland are the only countries to permit all five hormones sold on the international market.[35]

Animal feedstuff is not desirable, since the MAFF gave approval in 1985 for chicken litter – 'the bedding, faecal droppings, feathers and wasted food that is swept from poultry pens' to be used to feed beef cattle.[36] 'This type of feed is still in use' says a spokesperson for MAFF, 'but it is processed in accordance with statutory requirements. The process of waste products into food is subject to strict controls. It has been used for many years. The controls are obviously much stricter since the salmonella scare. I am sure there are many things we eat, that we would be surprised about if we knew their origins.' Cement dust, fed to cattle as a supplement, has been found to increase weight.[37] Methods such as these alter the fat/protein ratio. Animals reared in natural conditions, like wild animals, have a ratio which is healthy for man. Those reared quickly have an unhealthy ratio. EEC regulations have actually encouraged the breeding of animals with more fat in their meat and milk. Alternatively, they have encouraged the breeding of pigs with less fat, so that they cannot survive out of doors. Now, of course, the Milk Marketing Board is trying to sell milk with lower fat levels because saturated fat is seen as a health threat. (See Chapter 12.)

Slaughtering methods are usually stressful for the animal and this alters the flavour of the meat and, perhaps, its nutritional value. (If stress reduces nutrient levels in humans, it seems reasonable to suggest it can do the same in animals.)

Processing

The amount of processing depends on the final market product. Thus, some fruit and vegetables will be sold in the form in which it was harvested. However, some of it, especially apples and pears, will be subjected to some processing, such as waxing, to help it travel and store in 'good' condition. Storekeepers argue that the customer likes to see a shiny apple, equating this with quality. Do not be fooled! 'Perfect' foods, such as those sold by large retailers, can only be produced by the use of agrochemicals and careful marketing techniques.

The major purpose of most processing, however, is to add value. This does not mean 'nutritional value', but 'monetary value'. In fact, a good rule to apply is that the more monetary value added, the more nutritional value lost. The food industry is not abashed by this. As one newspaper report wrote of a leading meat producer: '...a more aggressive marketing strategy has resulted in record sales of *added value* turkey products... It is also considering withdrawing from pet food and other lines where it is difficult to *add value*'.[38] (Authors' italics.)

Many processed foods, cakes, biscuits, breads and 'sweets' are made from cheap ingredients and/or artificial ingredients, and therefore do not contain the level of nutrients in the home-made equivalent. You pay for what you get, and if an item is cheaper than the home-made version, it is usually because it is made from inferior ingredients, and is loaded with additives to disguise this.

Examples of processing include pulverising onions, then extruding them into onion shapes, coating them with breadcrumbs, cooking them and selling them frozen to restaurants. Fish which are small or whose name suggests they are inedible may be made into blocks and then cut into squares for fingers.[39]

When it comes to meat, the food technologists have produced a new range of products which is sold to the customer, legitimately, as 'meat'. Such products include Mechanically Recovered Meat, obtained by machines which strip flesh off bones. Meat, according to the 1984 Meat Products and Spreadable Fish Products Regulations, means 'the flesh, including fat, and the skin, rind, gristle and sinew in any amounts normally associated with the flesh used, of any animal or bird which is normally used for human consumption and includes any part of the carcass specified in Part 1 of Schedule 2 which is obtained from such an animal or bird, but does not include any other part of the carcass'.[40] Reformed meat may be shaped into 'steaks', or the poorest quality meats may be used in pies and other products.[41]

These are a few aspects of processing – we can only scratch the surface in this book. But before we leave the subject, let us look at some of the other major issues concerning it.

The value of whole grains

The 1983 report of the National Advisor Committee on Nutritional Education (NACNE) recommended increasing the amount of whole grains in the diet, not only because this would lead to an increase in dietary fibre, but also as it was 'more likely to ensure increased intakes of minerals, trace elements and other micronutrients; elemental malabsorption is also less likely'.[42] Why are whole grains a better food?

Taking wheat as an example, the question can be answered by considering what happens to the grains in the processing. The whole grain has three main parts: the outer layer, or bran; the germ; and the inner section, the endosperm. When the grain is milled to make white flour, the bran layer and 75 per cent of the germ are lost, leaving the flour consisting mostly of the endosperm.[43] But the parts lost contain most of the micronutrients needed by man, so large amounts of these are lost. As one expert wrote: '... the milling of refined white flour removes 40 per cent of the chromium, 86 per cent of the manganese, 76 per cent of the iron, 89 per cent of the cobalt, 68 per cent of the copper, 78 per cent of the zinc and 48 per cent of the molybdenum. 60 per cent of the calcium, 71 per cent of the phosphorus, 85 per cent of the magnesium, 77 per cent of the potassium, 78 per cent of the sodium...'[44] Valuable vitamins are lost also, among them being B1, B2, B3, B6, pantothenic acid, folic acid and E. B1 is particularly necessary for the metabolism of carbohydrates such as wheat and where it is absent in the food, the body will draw on its precious reserves from the central nervous system in order to metabolise the food for the energy it requires. Only a few of these vitamins are replaced in small amounts, each country having its own preferences. In addition, millers are required to add certain minerals. In Britain, for example, iron is added, though in a poorer form than that removed, and calcium, in the form of chalk, not a normal source of calcium. When the flour is later made into bread, various additives are also permitted, including bleaching agents, improvers, extenders and preservatives. Again, there is variation between countries.[45]

The dangers to health posed by this 'enriched' flour were demonstrated by Dr Roger Williams in an experiment with rats. He fed one group 'enriched' flour and another group the same flour but with many more added nutrients to make it similar to wholemeal. After 90 days, of the rats fed the 'enriched' flour 'about two-thirds were dead of malnutrition and the others were severely stunted'.[46]

Not only is white flour deficient of essential minerals, it may also contain high levels of cadmium. In its refining the zinc, which tends to be found in the bran layers, is lost, leaving the cadmium, found mostly in the centre of the grain. Cadmium is able to replace zinc in strategic enzymes and inactivate them.[47]

Some experts worry about a substance called phytate in flour, arguing that the phytate which is retained in wholemeal, but lost in the refining, binds up the zinc and carries it out of the body. The problem is compounded because the enzyme which destroys the phytate needs zinc. However, fermenting the bread with yeast increases the availability of zinc, because it seems to produce enzymes which destroy some of the phytate.[48] Unfortunately most bread today is not produced by fermenting yeast. Moreover, the practice of adding extra bran to the dough can further exacerbate zinc deficiency by adding extra phytate. Baking your own is the best way! You can also reduce the phytate in muesli by soaking the grains in water overnight.[49]

'Pure, White and Deadly'[50]

No, it is not the title of a thriller, but of a book by a world authority on sugar! This is his description of the substance which some doctors consider the most addictive there is.[51,52] Raw sugar, made from sugar cane juice by just evaporating the water content and allowing it to solidify and granulate, is dark brown and sticky, because of the molasses it contains.[53] These molasses are a rich source of trace elements which are necessary for the metabolism of sugar. When sugar cane or sugar beet is processed to give white sugar, all that remains is sucrose. Most of the trace minerals are lost, including '93 per cent of the chromium, 89 per cent of the manganese, 98 per cent of the cobalt, 98 per cent of the zinc and 98 per cent of the magnesium'.[54]

Physical methods of preserving foods

Man has preserved foods for centuries – and some of the methods are still in use, such as drying and salting. Once sugar was discovered to be a preservative it too became popular – just consider how much jam and marmalade is eaten! But advancing technology brought new methods, including freezing and canning. Food ceased to be preserved as a necessity in case of seasonal shortages. Tinned foods, and later on frozen ones, became cheap enough for everybody, often cheaper than fresh food, and with the advantage of a longer period of availability. With tinned peas, for example, you could eat them all year. What was overlooked was their inferior nutritional value. Freezing meat destroys 70 per cent of the pantothenic acid: in vegetables over half the B vitamins are lost. Canning is worse! Tinned peas and beans have lost over 75 per cent of pantothenic acid and Vitamin B6. For green vegetables the figure is over 50 per cent. Tinned tomatoes have had 80 per cent of their zinc removed, while carrots have lost 70 per cent of their cobalt. Storing the cans for a long time results in further losses of about 25 per cent.[55]

Food additives – the marvel of the food scientist!

Only a few decades ago, whatever the shortcomings of the food available, you could at least expect to be eating something that had either come out of the soil or was of animal, fish or bird origins. Not any longer! We now live in the era of the food scientist, who is not content with manufacturing a few colours or flavours – he actually makes 'foods' from his vast array of chemicals. Consider artificial sweeteners such as aspartame. Consider what happened to custard – changed from an egg dish to one made of cornflour and colourings. Consider what happened to a cup of lemon tea, which now contains dextrose, citric acid, soluble solids of tea, malto dextrin, acidity regulator (sodium citrate), natural lemon flavouring, Vitamin C, colouring (E102, E122, E132). Look at a packet of a raspberry flavour dessert and try to find where the raspberries are! No one can accuse the food scientists of idling over the last few decades. There are now about 4,000 additives in use in the UK, though only about 350 of them appear on labels.[56]

The 'E' numbers

Additives which have been reviewed by the EEC Scientific Committee on Food and deemed safe for wide use are given an 'E' which then appears in the list of ingredients. Do not assume that because they have been approved they are safe for you. Toxicological tests that the chemicals undergo do not reveal all the possible adverse effects nor are combinations of chemicals, as they appear in foods, subjected to testing. Other chemicals may be awaiting the Committee's consideration. Lastly, comparatively few additives are required to be listed. As two leading experts wrote: 'In reality, less than 10 per cent of all additives are ever listed on labels...At least 3,500 flavourings are used, and this entire class of chemicals is exempted from these labelling regulations. At most, a product may list "flavourings" on the label, but it is never stated whether one or 50 are being used, much less gives their names.'[57]

Not all additives are artificial, though this is not always understood in the general panic that has ensued over them in the media. Quite a few are derived from natural products, including some colours. Yet others are vitamins.

Not generally regarded as additives, but certainly the most common, are salt and sugar! In some foods, so much sugar is added that it becomes the main ingredient. You may not realise because it will be listed under different names: glucose, maltose, fructose, lactose, sucrose, dextrose and golden syrup, to mention but a few.[58]

If you are anxious to avoid them you can do this by buying fresh fruit, meat, fish, vegetables and grains, and doing your own baking. For other foods you can get good advice from books containing lists of additives, such as *Find Out*,[59] but these are only as helpful as the label on the food!

Irradiation

The Government is likely to decide it will permit some foods to be irradiated even though suitable tests to detect irradiation are not yet developed. However, we believe it is sufficiently harmful to include some information, since it is already permitted in a number of countries.

Food irradiation is a process by which food is exposed to high levels of gamma radiation to kill microscopic bacteria, thus increasing the shelf life of items such as grains, meat, herbs, spices, fruit and vegetables. Unless there is an error in the equipment or by the operator, the food does not become radioactive. However, electrons in the chemicals making up the food are knocked out of orbit and massive molecular rearrangement occurs. Free radicals are formed, the dangers of which were discussed in the last chapter. Vitamins A, D, C, E, K, B1, B2, B3, B6 and folic acid are depleted or destroyed. Some amino acids are broken down, fats go rancid, and carbohydrates create very toxic chemicals. New chemicals are formed called Unique Radiolytic Products (URPS), most being unknown and none has been adequately tested.

Irradiation will not make food safer – quite the reverse. It does not kill botulism, though it does kill botulism's natural enemies, thereby leaving the way open for botulism to thrive. Food which is 'off' will not have a warning smell. Other disease-producing organisms will be mutated, while aflatoxin, a highly carcinogenic compound produced by moulds, is produced in higher quantities. It does not reduce the use of chemicals in food, and no one knows what it does to their residues. In fact, it will increase the use of chemicals to counteract the changes in texture, smell and flavour produced as a result of the process. The British Medical Association is firmly opposed, arguing that it could put children's health at risk. Where animals have been fed irradiated foods adverse effects have included tumours, cataracts, chromosome breakage, kidney damage, fewer offspring and higher mortality.[60–62]

Do not believe the propaganda that this is a desirable process. Just as organophosphates were produced as the outcome of the weapons industry after the Second World War, so this is the result of a technology designed to use radioactive wastes from the nuclear industry.

Packaging and marketing of food products

In the battle to win the market for a food, the product is designed throughout by public relations experts in addition to the food scientist. As important as the ingredients – the PR people would argue more important – is the packaging and advertising. Enormous sums are spent on developing a new product, so nothing can be left to chance. In very inferior foods, the packaging may cost as much as the ingredients! Yet again, the emphasis is on profit, not health, with no concerns about the worries that some wrappings can have adverse effects. These include aluminium containers and coverings, and clingfilm, the chemicals of which can sometimes transmigrate to the food. Always look for paper bags and cellophane wrappers.

Food preparation

We have considered some aspects of this in chapter 5. Here we are concentrating on the decision on whether to cook or eat raw food.

Many famous doctors and naturopaths have advocated the benefits of raw foods, including Max Bircher-Benner, Max Gerson, Kristine Nolfi, John Douglass, as well as our three pioneers (see Chapter 5), most of them recommend a diet comprising 75 per cent raw food and 25 per cent cooked. Why do so many of them believe that 'cooking may damage your health'?[63] There are many reasons quoted, only some of which we can list:

- Cooking destroys vitamins. For example, if you cook fresh peas for five minutes, you destroy 20–40 per cent of Vitamin B1 and 30–40 per cent of Vitamin C.[64]
- Cooking destroys enzymes. These are essential for the efficient metabolism of food.[65] For example, the phosphatases in milk which break down the phosphorus-containing compounds, 'are

destroyed when milk is pasteurised. The result is that most of the calcium milk contains becomes insoluble, making milk constipating.'[66]
- Other proteins are deformed, with some of the amino acids being destroyed, while others may be altered so they are useless.[67]
- Fats heated to high temperatures change their structure from the 'cis' type, which the body needs and uses, to the 'trans' type, which the body cannot use, and which can cause harm to health.[68]

But not all foods can be eaten raw: cooking does have some advantages.
- It destroys harmful organisms, especially in meat, poultry and some shellfish.
- It breaks down toxins in red and black beans.
- It changes the tough connective tissues in meat to gelatin, making eating easier.
- You can eat more cooked food than raw – perhaps not an advantage if you are overweight!

Balance seems to be the key, with plenty of raw food in a varied diet.

Microwave ovens

Microwave ovens 'cook' food not by the application of heat to it, but by generating heat from within it.[65] If you must use one, do not stand near it when it is on; do not cover food with plastic to cook; remember that we know that microwaves affect cells, though we do not yet know if this can be harmful. On the other hand, no one has proved it is safe! (See Chapter 10.)

Conclusions

In this chapter we have explained how food production techniques can inhibit the provision of a healthy diet for the nation, including prospective parents and children. The best insurance you have against harmful methods is an organic wholefood diet, with appropriate nutritional supplements.

CHAPTER 12

Food-related Illness

HELP TO MINIMISE THE CHANCES OF ALLERGIC ILLNESS IN YOUR BABY.

Although we have conquered many serious infectious conditions, we are now seeing an escalation of diet-related diseases. There have, for example, been increases in the incidence of allergic illness, anorexia/bulimia and mental disorders. In this chapter, we examine some of the conditions that are diet-related and which have relevance to pregnancy. We are being very selective, for reasons of space, but any condition that affects the health of either prospective parent before conception, or the woman during pregnancy, may have adverse consequences for the outcome. Diabetes, for example, is known to be linked with difficult pregnancies, and diabetics are carefully monitored throughout though the orthodox approach might not be to alleviate the diabetes by adjustment of minerals before conception, as the Foresight doctor does. Here we concentrate on those illnesses that experience has shown are most common in people having problems with pregnancy, and which have tended to be overlooked in many cases, namely, allergies, coeliac condition, anorexia/bulimia and postnatal depression.

Allergy

In 1906 Clement von Pirquet, a pioneer in the study of immunisation, defined allergy as 'observable altered reactions to environmental substances'.[1] Unfortunately, as more research was done on allergy, allergists split into two camps: those who believed the answers lay in closely studying the immune system and those who were more concerned with considering a wider perspective.

Immunologists had discovered that when a foreign body enters the blood, the host body produces special protein substances called antibodies, which circulate in the blood and bind with the foreign body to neutralise it. An allergic person produces more antibodies than is necessary, and these irritate various tissues, causing a range of conditions, including asthma, eczema and hay fever. Immunologists can check for four types of reaction, using blood tests. If one or more is not positive, then allergy is said not to be present.

However, only a minority of people are found to have symptoms which fit this diagnosis. What about the many others who experience 'observable altered reactions'? Even now, some doctors will use the following logic: since it is not allergy and other tests reveal nothing, the symptoms must clearly not exist. They must, therefore, be imaginary. The patient is neurotic, a hypochondriac, a nuisance!

Not all doctors trod the immunologists' path. There were still some who continued to follow through the ideas of Francis Hare, a British psychiatrist who wrote a book in 1906 called *The Food Connection*.[2] But they were few, and they failed to convince the medical establishment of their ideas, so that today most of them are found in private practice, their work not often encouraged within the NHS.

Some doctors decide on new approaches and theories on the basis of studies they read in medical journals. Yet we saw in Chapter 7 that even reputable journals sometimes publish very bad research. This has also happened in the field of allergy. Many research projects assume that if there is no quick reaction to a test, allergy is not present. In food allergy this may be quite erroneous. Sometimes a person may not react to a food for many hours, even days. In a critical analysis of a study reported in the *Lancet*,[3] Jennifer Masefield has highlighted some of the study's weaknesses:[4]

> Dried encapsulated foods used for double-blind provocation tests may not give accurate results, because the actual state of the food may be the important factor. Some people can tolerate cooked cabbage but react to raw cabbage. The preparation of food can alter the allergen.
>
> Often certain food reactions are only caused by food combinations, so testing of foods in isolation will not produce a reaction.
>
> If an allergic person has not been exposed to an allergen for a long period he/she may have lost sensitivity to it. However, reactions may return after repeated exposures. In a multiple allergic patient who is repeatedly changing his/her diet to maintain better health, the sensitivity swing will make food allergy tests give different responses at different phases of the sensitivity level, for each excluded allergen or ingested allergen. This can give very confusing results, leading to an assumption of psychosomatic illness. If an allergen is excluded for only a few days, sensitivity is initially heightened and will show on testing.

At least two states in the USA have passed laws requiring examination for undiagnosed organic conditions either causing or exacerbating psychiatric symptoms.[5] Many studies are now linking allergy with conditions such as migraine, epilepsy and hyperactivity.[6,7,8] Self-help groups are increasing in number, and more doctors are becoming interested.

Relevance in preconception care

Foresight clinicians pay special attention to allergy for a number of reasons:
- If a prospective parent is suffering from a food allergy, health is impaired, and there may be malabsorption which will generally lead to nutritional deficiencies.

- Allergies in either prospective parent seem to lead to allergies in their offspring, which can seriously impair development.
- Clearing up allergies may mean that drugs do not need to be taken to alleviate the symptoms caused by the allergens.
- Allergies may cause excessive mucus which can lead to blocked Fallopian tubes, which cause infertility.
- If the mother's allergies are not resolved and she is breastfeeding, she may find her baby suffering, e.g. from colic from a masked cow's milk allergy in the mother.

Investigating allergy
There are a number of ways of investigating allergy, with varying degrees of effectiveness. We list below some of the main ones:
1. The clinical history is most important and, ideally, should include reference to the wider family, especially parents. (See Chapter 4.) Allergic symptoms may have been present early in life, may alter and not be diagnosed as the cause of later problems found in, for example, the hyperactive, learning disabled child, the delinquent teenager, and/or the aggressive husband who abuses his wife and children.
2. Questionnaires can be useful in identifying symptoms. We give an example in Appendix Three. As you can see, the list of symptoms is extensive. Indeed, it is this very wide range which makes some doctors so sceptical, and the investigation so difficult.
3. Bryan Cytotoxic blood tests, performed by skilled technicians, are approximately 75 per cent reliable for *food* allergy only, so can give useful guidance.
4. Skin prick tests and sublingual testing, which are sometimes used, are unreliable for food allergy.
5. Miller Provocation testing, a form of skin test, is more reliable and can be used to establish dosage for treatment.
6. Elimination and rotation diets are the most reliable methods. Many doctors specialising in ecological medicine (sometimes called clinical ecology or environmental medicine) put patients on a special diet to check for allergies. Depending on what the clinical history and questionnaires have revealed, it may mean cutting out all dairy produce and cereals, including refined carbohydrates. Basically this means eating meat and vegetables and the more unusual fruits such as pears. But not all meat and vegetables may be allowed. Often the patient will be asked to eat just lamb and game to start with if it is suspected that beef, pork and/or poultry may be allergens.

Easier than this is just eliminating one food group and noting the effects. This is often tried with the major allergens, which tend to be the foods/drinks most commonly ingested in a country, such as wheat, yeast, chocolate, tea, coffee, eggs and milk in the UK.

If this does not improve the situation you may wish to try a rotation diet, designed to give each specific food only one day in, say, five or seven days. The following rotation diet has worked well with many

Foresight patients. It should be used in conjunction with a food diary, in which every food and drink taken is noted, with the time. There should be a separate column for comments, which will include any effects felt, either physical or emotional, and the time they were experienced. This is very important, since we have said that the reaction may not be immediate. Remember, you are going to have to play detective, so you want all the evidence you can collect. (You may first wish to try the diary without the rotation diet.)

A rotation diet for the detection of allergy[9]

MONDAY	TUESDAY	WEDNESDAY	THURSDAY
Chicken	Pork	Lamb	Turkey
Banana	Sago	Brown rice	Maize (sweetcorn)
Pineapple	Dates	Rice flour	Cornflour
Beetroot	Apple	Orange	Leeks
Spinach	Pear	Grapefruit	Onions
Swiss chard	Lettuce	Satsuma	Asparagus
Pineapple juice	Endive	Mandarin	Chives
	Chicory	Lime	Grapes
	Artichoke	Carrot	Sultanas
	Sunflower seeds	Celery	Grape juice
	Apple juice	Parsnip	
		Parsley	
		Orange or grapefruit juice	

FRIDAY	SATURDAY	SUNDAY
Fish	Rabbit	Beef
Millet	Lentils	Potato
Millet flakes	Green beans	Potato flour
Cabbage	Peas	Tomato
Savoy cabbage	Blackeyed beans	Aubergine
Brussels sprouts	Broad beans	Cucumber
Broccoli	Mung bean shoots	Marrow
Cauliflower	Plums	Melon
Kohlrabi	Peaches	Tomato juice
Swedes	Apricot	
Avocado	Cherry	
Figs	Prunes	
Water	Prune juice	

A word of warning: whatever type of diet you try, be it elimination or rotation, when you come off an allergen you are usually going to suffer some sort of withdrawal symptoms that will make you feel worse. It may be similar to having a hangover, as you are often addicted to the foods to which you are allergic. Persevere, because you are going to feel better than ever once you are over the effects! It is probably wise to start your new diet when the next few days are free of pressure.

If you do find allergies, seek advice from one of the self-help organisations, a nutritionist who understands allergy, or a doctor who is experienced in nutritional medicine, to ensure that your diet and nutritional supplements provide all the nutrients you require. This is especially important if you are planning a pregnancy or are pregnant.

Do not despair! You will find there are many alternatives to our usual foods, which will add interest and variety to your diet. If you look in your local healthfood or wholefood store you will see many different types of flour, grains and milks. You may also find that your allergies change over time, although if you sort out your nutritional imbalances allergies sometimes become a thing of the past. Do not expect to be well if you only deal with your allergies and not other problems.

Always try to choose an organically grown food, free of additives. (See Chapter 5.)

The rotation diet is designed to give each specific food only one day in seven. The diet eliminates the most common allergens, cow's milk, grains and eggs. Also, all stimulants such as coffee, tea, chocolate and the sugars. No drink should be taken except the juice of the day and water. All foods must be boiled in plain water, steamed, plain grilled or cooked in the oven in a covered dish. No fats, oils, gravies are to be used. During the trial period NO FOOD OTHER THAN THOSE LISTED MAY BE TAKEN AT ALL.

During the first week of the diet adverse reactions may take place due to the withdrawal of cow's milk, etc, if these are allergic substances. For a few days the reactions may be quite strong, akin to alcohol withdrawal in the first few days of abstinence.

The food can be taken in various ways. Tuesday breakfast could be bacon slices; lunch a pork chop; the evening meal slices from a pork joint. On Wednesday breakfast could be lamb's kidneys; lunch could be a lamb chop and the evening meal could be lamb's liver. Beef could be alternated with veal, brains, ox-tail, ox-tongue, etc.

Unfinished food of the day should be put in the freezer for the following week. If not more fruit, veg, etc, is bought than will be consumed on the day, temptation will be removed for the following day. The participant may be more hungry than usual, however, and it is important to have enough food available.

The diet will have ensured a fast of six days from any offending food so the reaction to the allergen will probably be fairly immediate and may take the form of a running or stuffed-up nose, headache, stomach pain, feeling of bloatedness, extreme lethargy, irritability, etc. The day this occurs can be marked on the diet sheet. It is then possible to test the foods eaten on this day one at a time.

Having thus worked out a basic diet of 'safe' foods, it will then be possible to test common allergens, such as cow's milk, eggs, the gluten grains – wheat, oats, barley, rye – and other fruits, etc. After three weeks' abstinence the reaction may be strong, so at first only a small quantity of the substance should be given. If the reaction is very severe, a teaspoonful of bicarbonate of soda in water will help to alleviate the symptoms.

After an adverse reaction a return to known safe foods for a few days will be necessary before testing for another possible allergen. After a few weeks it should be possible to identify all food allergies in this way.

The treatment of food allergies will depend on a number of factors, including how extensive the allergies are. You may be able to get by with simple elimination, though this is no cure. There are various desensitising methods, ranging from drops to injections. The most practical and successful is probably enzyme potentiated desensitisation, though, as with all methods, it does not work for everyone.[10] Any doctor who is practising as a clinical ecologist, or using a nutritional approach in his work, will be able to diagnose and treat you. You will not be able to get desensitisation done except by a doctor.

Allergies to chemicals, such as food additives, pesticides and chemicals used in the workplace and home, may also be present. These are often difficult to diagnose and eliminate.[11]

Coeliac condition

This is a condition in which the sufferer cannot metabolise gluten, a protein found in wheat, barley, oats and rye. It can cause severe physical and mental symptoms if it is not diagnosed, mainly because of the severe deficiencies arising from the malabsorption. Coeliac conditions have been found to exacerbate infertility problems, especially in zinc deficient women. Treatment is by avoidance of gluten containing grains.

Malabsorption

Malabsorption is not a disease or illness in itself, but the result of other conditions such as allergies, infections, coeliac disease, candidiasis, nutritional deficiencies and toxic metal excesses, irritable bowel syndrome, Crohn's disease and colitis. Clearly, if you are not absorbing nutrients properly, you are likely to have nutritional deficiencies which can affect pregnancy outcome. Your hair analysis and other tests may reveal a malabsorption pattern. It is important that you seek medical help.

Anorexia/bulimia

Anorexia nervosa is often called 'the slimmer's disease', because it is thought that the sufferer stops eating because they are afraid of getting fat. In bulimia nervosa, the patient, usually older than the typical anorexic, may not eat for days and then binges, only to vomit the foods up, often in secret. The two conditions may lead to infertility because of low levels of essential nutrients, especially zinc. Even if infertility is not a problem, the anorexic or bulimic may put the fetus at risk because of these low levels. (We saw in Chapter 5 how underweight in the prospective mother could be disadvantageous.)

In 1984, Professor Bryce-Smith and Dr Simpson reported in the *Lancet* the first case of anorexia nervosa being successfully treated with zinc.[12] This condition had been classed as a psychiatric disorder. The recovery rate was not good – patients may have improved sufficiently to be out of danger, but many hovered in and out of anorexic states and some died. The usual patient is an adolescent girl, and it is this that has led to confusion, even to its being regarded as a situation in which the girl was afraid of growing up. Often the family have been seen as partly to blame, especially the parents. Treatment has been largely family therapy, drugs, forced feeding and behaviour therapy, in which rewards are linked to weight gain. Usually the weight was lost on release from hospital. Since weight gain was seen as the most important target, little or no attention was paid to nutritious food, the emphasis being on calories. This results in diets rich in refined carbohydrates (white sugar and white flour predominating in hospital food) and low in nutrients, a serious problem in any sick person, but of crucial importance if the condition is basically one of zinc, iron or magnesium deficiency. (It may also be relevant to consider the B vitamins and Vitamin E.) Some feminist writers believe anorexia is an attempt to cope in a world hostile to women. Others believe that eating is the only area in which the sufferer is able to exercise control over their life.[13] However, none of the theories has been proved, and it is difficult to understand how they have any credence.

It seems logical to assume that a disorder that is focused on eating will have some links with nutrition. Professor Bryce-Smith and his co-author, Liz Hodgkinson, have suggested that 'anorexia nervosa is basically a nutritional disorder resulting from greatly reduced food intake which may itself have social origins. This is combined, in susceptible people, with a probably inherited subnormal ability to utilize available zinc'.[14] (See Chapters 5, 7, 9, 11 and 15.) It all seems very reasonable – zinc is linked with the ability to smell and taste. If you are deficient, you will not enjoy food, as you will not taste or smell it properly. It is, therefore, not difficult to resist it. The less you have the more zinc deficient you become and the vicious circle spirals. You may suffer diarrhoea, further compounding the problem. The muscles become soft and flabby and may be misidentified as 'fat'.

Zinc is also necessary for proper brain functioning – if you are deficient you are likely to have the misperceptions that anorexics suffer. It is also vital for sexual and emotional maturity, both generally retarded in anorexics. The more one reviews the symptoms of anorexia, the more one is drawn to the conclusion that the zinc hypothesis is the most likely explanation. Of course, it does not apply to every case: Professor Bryce-Smith considers that maybe 15 per cent of patients do not improve,[15] but there could be many reasons for this, including failure to diagnose an oesophagal obstruction or infection.

There are a number of reasons why the zinc treatment should always be the *first* choice to be tried:
1. Unlike all the psychiatric measures, it does not cause harm. Of course, some counselling for patient and family may be beneficial,

as there is always considerable anxiety, but it should be completely non-judgmental, merely supportive. Drugs and electro-convulsive therapy always have severe side effects, and behaviour therapy is cruel if the problem is physical.
2. It can be given, without cruelty, even where the sufferer is uncooperative in treatment, since they do not need to know it is being given.
3. If a deficiency is the main problem, improvement, in most cases, will be rapid and the patient will not deteriorate too much before the treatment works.
4. It is easy to carry out the treatment at home.
5. It is cheap – costing less than the fare for a hospital visit in most cases.

How to check for and treat zinc deficiency
All you need to do to check your zinc status is buy a solution of zinc sulphate, now in the form of Zincatest from Nature's Best, or Check Zinc from the chemist, and follow the instructions. Your doctor can also get a supply from Lamberts. If there is a deficiency, supplement with drops from Cantassium or zinc citrate tablets from Nature's Best or Lamberts. (See Appendix One for addresses.) An initial supplement of 45–50 mg a day should show improvement in a week.[16]

○ WHAT IF THERE IS NO IMPROVEMENT? The problem may be iron or magnesium deficiency, in which case you can supplement with these, getting iron tablets from the chemist or using Epsom salts or milk of magnesia for magnesium.[17] Alternatively you can buy magnesium orotate and iron orotate tablets.

If there is no improvement after a few days, it is important to seek help from a doctor trained in nutrition, who can do biochemical and physical tests. If you have any drug treatment ensure that your nutritional status is closely monitored (see chapter 8).

Postnatal depression
Although we are focusing on postnatal depression, our comments apply, in general, to any form of depression. Most depression is organic (allergic)/biochemical in origin and should be investigated as a *physical disorder*.[18,19]

Postnatal depression always has serious consequences for the family: the mother does not get the pleasure from her baby that is her right; the baby does not get the benefit of a healthy mother, which may lead to feeding problems, and developmental problems; the husband and other children also suffer from a tired, sick wife and mother. Sometimes the depression is so severe the mother is hospitalised, thereby splitting the family. Sometimes she is even separated from her baby. If it is a first baby, the mother will feel inadequate, unable to cope, and may reluctantly decide not to have further children. Yet the situation need not arise!

Postnatal depression has many aspects to it, making it seem

complex. When the mother has given birth, she will have a high copper level, since copper is naturally raised at this time, and a low zinc level (remember animals eat the placenta, the richest source of zinc known). Giving birth may cause abrasions, which further deplete the body's zinc. She will be tired just from giving birth, and if she is in a noisy maternity ward, she may have problems sleeping. She will be regularly woken by her own baby. If she is zinc deficient, her milk will probably not contain sufficient quantities for her baby to thrive and he/she may cry a lot. If she is manganese deficient (and this is likely as one does not generally suffer from one deficient mineral) she may be confused and have difficulty organising herself at a time when she is having to adjust to many new activities. Zinc and manganese are factors in sugar metabolism, and deficiencies may lead to blood sugar swings, making the feelings of fatigue worse.

In all cases of depression, vitamin and mineral supplements will prove helpful. Remember that if drugs are given, they will always have side effects, including causing nutritional imbalances. The first action should be a nutritional approach. (See Chapter 5.)

Depression is very rare in mothers who have followed the Foresight programme, probably because their nutritional status is good throughout the pregnancy.

Lactation problems

There is no doubt that 'Breast is Best!' When the baby is born the first liquid taken from the breast is colostrum, which is rich in antibodies, essential fats and zinc. This is vital for the baby's immature immune system and is the reason why colostrum should always be the first substance ingested by the baby. It is widely known that babies who are put on formula feeds from birth often develop allergies to cow's milk protein.[20] Human milk is also rich in antibodies and all the nutrients the baby needs to develop properly, especially if the mother is healthy. Even though there have been reports that breast milk has high levels of pesticides and other toxins, since these are obtained from foods ingested by the mother, they are also likely to be present in food used for baby foods, since they are not prepared from organically produced foods. (Of course, the Foresight mother eating organic food will be ingesting a lower level of pesticides anyway.)

Lactation problems can cause major misery for mother and child. The hungry baby will cry and fail to thrive at a time when his developing brain needs good nutrition. Too little milk may lead to supplementing with formula feeds, which can only approximate human milk. Nipples in a mother who has nutritional deficiencies may be sore, making feeding difficult. What should be a rewarding experience for mother and baby becomes painful.

Conclusion

Most disease has some dietary aspect and will respond, at least in part, to nutritional intervention and the removal of toxins. This is especially true of the disorders discussed, although it is not widely recognised. Our general advice for any condition must be to consider how nutrition can help alleviate some/all of the symptoms. This applies even in situations of accident, since any trauma to the body, such as a broken limb, internal injuries, or open wounds, cause stress to the body and this depletes nutrients, especially zinc, Vitamin C and Vitamin E.

CHAPTER 13

Diseases

HELP WITH HOW TO RECOGNISE AND ELIMINATE INFECTIONS PRIOR TO CONCEPTION — AND WHY YOU NEED TO DO SO.

We have long recognised that certain diseases can adversely affect the fetus (e.g. German measles), or cause sterility (e.g. mumps). But we often overlook the importance of genito-urinary infections, which include sexually transmitted diseases. Clearly, any infection in the baby at the start of its life is serious. We have seen that stress increases the need for nutrients — nutrients which are needed for the development of the sperm, egg or fetus. Thus, infection can indirectly affect development. It may, of course, have direct effects, causing sight problems (eye infections) or brain damage (as in some meningitis cases).

In this chapter we review some of the literature on the most serious conditions, especially the genito-urinary infections. (We omit infections such as malaria and tuberculosis, since these are not common in the UK.)

German measles (rubella)

This is not usually serious for the adult, but for the fetus it can have grave consequences. The dangers of abnormalities are about 50 per cent in the first few weeks of pregnancy, about 17 per cent in the third month, and almost 0 per cent thereafter. Some of the effects include congenital cataracts, deafness, heart disease, microcephaly, stunted growth, malformation of the teeth and low birth weight. There may also be miscarriages.[1]

It would seem that there may be cumulative effects during life, if the fetus is exposed to infection. In a study of 3,076 people who had been exposed, some of whom were 40 years old at the time of the investigation, the results confirmed a cumulative incidence of deafness to at least 15 per cent by the age of 20 years.[2]

Chickenpox and shingles

These are caused by the herpes varicella-zoster virus. Problems are rare, because most women have established immunity to the virus, and because the virus does not tend to cross the placenta. However, in a very small number of babies born to women who do become infected, there seems to be a distinct pattern, including prematurity, skin lesions, neurologic anomalies, eye anomalies, skeletal abnormalities, gastro-intestinal and genito-urinary anomalies.[3] Infections early in pregnancy may also lead to prematurity, stillbirth or abortion.[4] Other research has noted reduction and deformity of limbs, low birth weight and meningoencephalitis.[5] High tone deafness occurred in one child, where the mother had been infected at 38 weeks gestation.[6]

Toxoplasmosis

This is an infection which may result from eating raw meat and raw fish, or from contact with cats or cat litter. If it is contracted in the first half of pregnancy, it may cause hydrocephalus, eye problems, psychomotor retardation, convulsions, microphthalmia, and intracerebral calcifications (calcium deposits in the brain). In the second half of pregnancy, the damage it may cause to the fetus is likely to be less severe.[7]

Cytomegalovirus (CMV)

Caused by one of the herpes viruses, this can have serious problems for men, women and infants. It is linked with low sperm count and inflammation of the testicle.[8] Prenatally, it can cause miscarriage. Some 3,000 babies are estimated to be infected each year, 300 of them being left with a subsequent handicap.[9] It is the most commonly known viral cause of mental retardation, though it may also be responsible for other conditions.[10] These include microcephaly, psychomotor retardation, developmental abnormalities[11] and progressive hearing impairment,[12] respiratory illness, jaundice, small size for gestational age, failure to thrive and eye infections.[13]

Mumps

For the fertile male, mumps can cause inflammation of the various parts of the sex organs, leading to eventual sterility in some cases. But it can also affect the fetus. An excess of diabetes was found among people exposed to the infection in the mother's womb in the first three months of pregnancy. By the age of 30 years, researchers had found a 15-fold increased risk of developing diabetes.[14]

Genito-urinary infections

Sadly, the number of people suffering from genito-urinary problems continues to rise to what some doctors consider epidemic proportions.[15] There are many reasons – increased use of the pill and IUD, poor nutritional status, leading to a weak immune system, and earlier sexual activity, to mention but a few. Greater sexual freedom, leading to more partners, has certainly increased the risk of infections, though some genito-urinary conditions occur even among couples who are completely faithful to each other (e.g.

candidiasis). Most of the infections can have dire consequences for fertility, sterility, and the fetus, not to mention the general health of the sufferer. We have not explained the symptoms of the various conditions, because they are not always apparent. If, however, you think there is any chance, whatsoever, that you may have an infection, especially if you have an unpleasant or coloured discharge, you should tell your doctor. Your preconception care should include any appropriate check-up and treatment. (See Chapter 4.)

Common sexually transmitted diseases

VIRUSES	Wart (HPV)
	Herpes
	Cytomegalovirus*
	Hepatitis B*
	AIDS*
MYCOPLASMAS	Mycoplasma hominis*
	Ureaplasma urealyticum*
BACTERIA	Chlamydia trachomatis
	Gonorrhoea
	E. coli*
	Entercocci
	B. streptococci
	Gardenella
	Bacteroides ⎫
	Mixed anaerobes ⎬ Anaerobes
	Syphilis ⎭

The only normal vaginal bacteria known is Lactobacillus.

FLAGELLATES	Trichomonas
FUNGI	Candida – thrush*

* Indicates the condition is not exclusively sexually transmitted in adults.
Adapted from Grant, Ellen. Unpublished, 1988.

Candidiasis (thrush)

The yeast, candida albicans, occurs naturally in the body, and in healthy people it causes no problems. It is well known as the cause of thrush, both oral, which is common in babies, and vaginal. But it is now recognised that an overgrowth of the yeast can be a contributory factor in many other conditions.[16,17] In some cases this may arise as a condition secondary to viral or bacterial infections which thrive because of a weakened immune system. The use of antibiotics kills off both good and bad organisms in the gut and other mucous membranes, allowing the yeasts, which are not killed off, to proliferate. Symptoms of chronic candidiasis are many. Those such as allergies and sensitivity to food and/or chemicals, craving for refined carbohydrates and/or alcohol, and alcohol intolerance, irritable bowel syndrome, iron or zinc deficiency can affect nutritional status and may therefore compromise reproductive outcomes (though, as we have said before, any symptom which shows an adverse state of health could do this).[18] One authority has said that there was a doubling of new cases of genital candidiasis reported between 1971 and 1975.[19] Such candidiasis may also cause painful intercourse and possibly provide a hostile environment for the sperm. With treatment, which includes anti-fungal agents and nutritional therapy, most of the symptoms can be relieved. Short courses of Vitamin A, which protects the mucous membranes, have been found to be helpful, as has the local application of yoghourt. (You should take a maximum of up to 21,000 IUs for three to four days, reducing to 7,000 IUs. This should be reduced to 2,000 IUs before conception. The larger dose should be taken during menstruation to be certain pregnancy has not occurred.)

Chlamydia

Chlamydia trachomatis is a nasty pathogen (disease-carrying organism) which is thought to be the most common sexually transmitted pathogen in the Western industrialised world. It is responsible for a great deal of sexually transmitted infection, as well as infertility, and ill health in infants.[20] Since the symptoms are not always obvious, the woman may not even realise she has it, until her health is very much undermined.

In men, chlamydia, as it is usually called, causes between one-third and a half of non-gonococchal urethritis, although it often occurs together with gonorrhoea.[21] It can also cause inflammation of the prostate tubes, a painful and potentially sterilising infection, or even of the rectum, testes and *vas deferens*, and other complicated genital infections.

In women, it is a major cause of pelvic inflammatory disease (see below), cervicitis, cervical cell dysplasia and urethral syndrome.[22] When it spreads from the cervix to the womb lining, it may induce endometriosis.[23] If it goes on to the Fallopian tubes,[24] it can cause salpingitis, which can result in blocked tubes and infertility.[25] If the tubes are partially blocked there is a risk of an ectopic pregnancy, which can be very serious. More antibodies are found in infertile couples than in fertile ones.[26]

In children, at least 50 per cent of infants born to chlamydia positive women are likely to develop infections.[27] One study quoted a 61 per cent rate of infection, with a 44 per cent rate of clinical disease in infants born to infected mothers.[28] Prematurity may result, and other main problems are conjunctivitis, found in 25–50 per cent of exposed infants, and pneumonia in 10–20 per cent.[29] Rhinitis, otitis media, proctitis and vulvitis have also been reported. For example, in one study, exposed infants had twice the rate of pneumonitis and recurrent otitis media in their first six months of life. Those who had pneumonitis had higher subsequent rates of gastroenteritis. The researchers concluded: 'These results suggest that appreciable outpatient infant mortality may be associated with maternal infection with chlamydia trachomatis and that it may either cause or promote the occurrence of early recurrent otitis media and gastroenteritis.'[30] Another study found chlamydia trachomatis in the infant's pharynx and conjunctiva, the mother's cervix and the father's urethra. The researchers recommended searching for chlamydial infections in preterm infants with atypical respiratory disease even if delivered by caesarian section.[31]

Gonorrhoea

Caused by the bacteria, *Neisseria gonorrhoea-gonococcus*, this is one of the most contagious diseases there is. Often the symptoms pass unnoticed, but if it is not treated, it can have very serious consequences for men, women and infants.

In men it can lead to sterility and low sperm counts. In the female, it is a major cause of pelvic inflammatory disease, which may lead to sterility. It also seems to leave her more vulnerable to chlamydial infections.[32]

If a woman has suffered from gonorrhoea, she is likely to be tested during pregnancy (though with good preconception care, she should be free from infection before conceiving). At least one researcher has found that prolonged rupture of the membranes and later chorioamniocentesis in infected women predisposes the baby to acquire the infection.[33] There are also risks of prematurity in infected women.[34]

Infections in the newborn are common if the mother is infected, as the bacteria are passed to the baby during its passage through the birth canal. Conjunctivitis is the most common problem, as the conjunctiva come into contact with the infected cervix during birth – this can lead to a serious discharge with risks to sight, including blindness.[35] Other parts of the body may also suffer, with infections of the umbilicus, the anogenital area, or nose and throat. There may be arthritis or meningitis.[36]

Herpes

There are various types of herpes virus, causing a number of conditions, some of which we have already mentioned. However, it is the herpes simplex virus which causes the condition known commonly as 'herpes'. There are two similar types – Type 1 causes sores around the mouth and nose, often referred to as 'cold sores', and, more rarely, in the eyes or genital or anal area. Type 2 causes sores in the genital and anal area and, more rarely, on the mouth. Genital infections caused by Type 2 are the more severe. Small sores appear which can be quite painful. There may be itching or pain on urinating. The symptoms clear but further attacks may occur.[37]

It is very important for a woman to tell her doctor if she has or has had genital herpes as it could affect the birth procedure. A caesarian section may be advised where there is an active sore in the vagina or on the cervix.[38] If the waters break, a path is created for the virus to reach the baby, so a caesarian section should be done quickly.[39] The virus may also be passed to the baby after birth by kissing if one has a cold sore or if there are sores on the breasts during breastfeeding. It is rare for the fetus to be infected in the womb and this would generally result in a miscarriage.[40]

Researchers have concluded that herpes 'can result in spontaneous abortion, congenital and perinatal infections in the infant, or disseminated infection and death in the mother'. The frequency of risk factors is unknown. In their study there was a 40 per cent incidence of serious perinatal disease or illness. Some of the infants whose mothers became infected in the last three months of pregnancy had perinatal morbidity such as prematurity, intrauterine growth retardation, and neonatal infections with herpes Type 2.[41]

A main problem is that the baby's immature system may not be able to cope with the virus and this can lead to an overwhelming infection, resulting in encephalitis with consequent brain damage, or eye infections, with eye damage. There may be jaundice, pneumonia with breathing difficulties, or even spells with no breathing at all. Microcephaly, microphthalmia and intracranial calcification have also been reported.[42] There have been reports of physical impotence in men who suffered from herpes and proctitis, which then resulted in nerve inflammation.[43]

Syphilis

This is a very dangerous infection if it is not treated, though fortunately it responds to *early* treatment. In both sexes it can lead to sterility, and damage to many vital organs, including the heart and brain. The brain damage leads to psychiatric problems.

Syphilis is transmitted from the mother to the fetus via the placenta, thus making it prenatal rather than congenital, though in the child it is usually referred to as 'congenital syphilis'. It only occurs when the mother's syphilis is not diagnosed and treated, making it now comparatively rare as most women's blood is screened at the antenatal stage.[44] (Of course, if you have followed the Foresight programme you will be screened before conception.)

Without treatment one third of the babies will be born healthy, one third will be aborted or stillborn, and one third will have congenital syphilis. Stillbirths will occur if the maternal infection is present very early in pregnancy and if there is so great a dose of the organism responsible that the fetus succumbs to infection.[45]

The baby suffering from congenital syphilis may appear healthy at birth, though occasionally there may be a rash. However, failure to thrive and gain weight, often the first clinical signs of early congenital syphilis, become apparent two to eight weeks after birth. There may be weight loss, and often the baby has a wizened appearance, like an old man. Other symptoms include skin lesions, mucous membrane lesions, visceral lesions, enlarged liver and/or spleen, abdominal swelling, meningitis, and bone lesions.[46]

Mycoplasmas, including ureaplasma urealyticum

These organisms are the smallest free-living pathogens, capable of causing a wide range of problems in humans. In the reproductive system, mycoplasma hominis and ureaplasma urealyticum are the most commonly cultured. A direct relation between the frequency of venereal infection and serum antibody levels has been found.[47] One authority writes: 'Mycoplasmas, which commonly reproduce when the subject's health is impaired, can cause attacks of vulvovaginitis, genital irritation and urinary frequency. Symptoms may persist for twenty years or even longer.'[48]

In men, ureaplasma urealyticum is a major cause of non-gonococcal urethritis, which can lead to infertility,[49] non-specific urethritis (NSU), prostate and kidney disease.[50] High concentrations have been found in the genital tracts of sterile couples than in fertile couples.[51] In women, pelvic inflammatory disease can result if the mycoplasmas, including ureaplasma urealyticum, are allowed to proliferate. Scarring may lead to infertility. (See Chapter 9 also.) Miscarriage and premature birth are also associated with them.[52] Of the common organisms ureaplasma urealyticum is the most frequently implicated in repetitive abortions.[53]

Genital mycoplasma infection is difficult to eradicate and prospective parents who have such a condition may have to be patient.[54] Women need local treatment of the cervix.

Pelvic inflammatory disease

This has already been mentioned. (See sections on chlamydia, gonorrhoea and mycoplasmas.) It can be gonococcal, chlamydial, or non-gonococcal, non-chlamydial in type. It is sometimes misdiagnosed so that tests for all types should always be conducted. Treatment for one type may be ineffective against another. For example, antibiotics for gonorrhoea do not cure chlamydia.[55] One study found a high incidence of non-gonococcal infection among the male partners of women with PID. Over three-quarters of the males were showing no symptoms.[56]

The consequences of untreated PID are severe – they may include sub-fertility, sterility, menstrual difficulties, chronic abdominal pain and ectopic pregnancy.[57] The risks of tubal infection leading to infertility seem to be related to the number and types of infection. In one study, even after treatment with antibiotics, a single tubal infection, including chlamydia, produced a 12.8 per cent infertility rate, two infections produce a 35.5 per cent infertility rate, while for three it is a 75 per cent rate.[58] Catterall reports, in respect of an infection of both gonorrhoea and chlamydia, that: 'If the statistics are correct there is a 50 per cent chance of relapse..., a one in three chance of being sterile, a 25 per cent chance of dyspareunia (painful intercourse) and a 10 per cent chance of an ectopic pregnancy'.[59]

Genital warts – condyloma accuminata

These are caused by a virus called 'papilloma virus'. The symptoms may only be warty nodules which may not be readily apparent. Some types of the virus have been linked with cervical cancer and may therefore affect reproduction.[60] By 1987, one in six women attending

Islington family planning clinics had a positive smear. One in three had either cell abnormalities and/or the cancer wart-virus.[61] (It is not clear, though, how representative a group this is, compared with the general population.)

Trichomoniasis

This condition is caused by the organism trichomonas. Women may suffer from excessive (itchy) vaginal discharge, while the newborn may have fever, irritability and may fail to thrive.[62]

Hepatitis B

Hepatitis means 'inflammation of the liver'. Type B, one of three types, can be spread through sexual contacts or contact with body fluids, such as blood, urine and saliva, so it is not just sexually transmitted. Like chlamydia and gonorrhoea, it is possible to have it without any symptoms. Treatment may be slow, being bed rest and nutritional therapy. Vaccination is available to some people, although at least one authority has advocated screening for everyone, with vaccination as appropriate, because it is a serious condition leading to neonatal deaths.[63] It can also lead to an increase in food and chemical sensitivities in the mother, which may affect a baby who is being breastfed.[64]

AIDS – Acquired Immune Deficiency Syndrome

Although the subject of much public debate, AIDS is still quite rare, though its incidence is increasing quickly. The main way that the virus which causes it (HIV) is transmitted is by sexual activity, either hetero- or homo-. A few people have been infected by contaminated blood transfusions and some drug addicts by infected needles.

Although some treatments, aimed at strengthening the immune system, may sometimes arrest progress of the condition. Women who have antibodies of the virus in your blood you should not become pregnant, as it is known that pregnancy will increase the risk of developing AIDS. Moreover, babies born to HIV infected mothers have a high chance of being infected whole in the womb. They are then prone to infections in life, with a reduced quality of life and reduced life expectancy.

Conclusions

Many infections can be damaging, either to the reproductive tract, the sperm, ova, or fetus. We have written about the most common infections individually, but unfortunately they often occur in combination, and this multiplies the risks of damage. In one study, mycoplasma hominis was found in 30–50 per cent of vaginal cultures of sexually active women, with ureaplasma urealyticum in 60–80 per cent of cultures.[65] Another study looked at the incidence of six infections in pregnant adolescents. They were aged 13–17 years, all from very poor socio-economic backgrounds and in their third trimester. The results showed that only five appeared to be free from all the infections being considered, while 34 per cent had trichimonas, 38 per cent candidiasis, 70 per cent mycoplasma homini and 90 per cent ureaplasma urealyticum. Chlamydia trachomatis was found in 37 per cent of 105 specimens. Gonorrhoea was originally present in 12 subjects early in pregnancy, but only in one in the third trimester. In addition, three had evidence of genital herpes infection and three others evidence of papovirus infection.[66]

While the immune system may cope with one mild infection, if there are multiple infections, it is likely to be unable to withstand such an onslaught, thus increasing the risks of damage. There is also the risk that not all infections will be treated, even if symptoms persist. Comprehensive screening is vital and it is sensible that, where possible, a colposcope should be used as it is a superior technique for at least one condition[67] and thought to be a better technique for others.[68] If you suspect that you may have an infection, ask your doctor for a full examination with the appropriate swabs taken and the use of a colposcope. This may mean travelling a bit, as, according to one doctor's survey, fewer than half of the UK's genito-urinary clinics have unlimited access to a chlamydia diagnostic service, half offer a restricted service, and eight cannot test at all.[69] Very few doctors have access to a colposcope and of those, few are looking for mycoplasmas. However, in view of the many adverse effects of genito-urinary infections, it is worth making an effort to get the best treatment available. Any infections or cell abnormalities on the cervix should be diagnosed and treated before pregnancy as the rise in hormones during pregnancy increases these problems. The extra hormone stimulation given to infertile women is especially likely to cause a flare-up of cervical or pelvic infection.[70]

Checklist

1. Have you had your rubella status checked?
2. Avoid eating raw meat and fish. Wash cats' dishes separately. Do not allow cats on cooking surfaces. If you are pregnant, do not handle soiled cat litter.
3. Ask for a genito-urinary examination if you suspect an infection or if you are having difficulty in conceiving. For a woman this should involve the use of a colposcope.
4. Remember that barrier methods of contraception, the condom and the diaphragm, have been found to give some protection against infections, including tubal infections.[71]
5. If a genito-urinary infection is diagnosed it is vital that both partners receive treatment and follow-up checks.
6. The male partner should have the semen and/or the prostatic fluid checked for infection. Urine screening alone is adequate.

CHAPTER 14

Tests During Pregnancy

TESTS YOU MAY BE INVITED TO UNDERGO DURING PREGNANCY — THE PROS AND CONS.

When you are pregnant you will be given a variety of tests. Some are quite routine and will be done on most antenatal checks. These include blood and urine tests and blood pressure. They are made mainly to check that your health is not a threat to the baby. But now, with modern medical technology, you may be offered others which monitor the health of your baby, looking for genetic disorders and congenital abnormalities. It is these that we examine in this chapter. The tests should be supportive of genetic counselling, not a substitute for it, although there is a trend for them to be offered as routine. For example, many women are now offered a scan, without any specific reason for it. Indeed, it has been argued that scans should be done in every pregnancy as a precaution.[1,2] All tests should be given careful thought: it is perhaps ironical that the tests are especially recommended in high risk pregnancies when most of them carry risks in themselves! If, therefore, you can minimise your chances of having any test, you should do so. The information in this chapter will help you both with the decision – remember, it is yours to make.

Deciding whether or not to have the tests

Not everyone will be offered all the tests. They need careful thought, ideally before the pregnancy, as it is difficult to be objective during it, especially if, in the event of an unfortunate outcome, you have to contemplate an abortion. They should be considered only when there is an increased risk of severe genetic disorder or birth defect for which there is little or no effective treatment, such as in Down's syndrome or neural tube defects. The risks of the tests should be defined and attitudes to abortion should be discussed. Family history may indicate other risks, such as haemophilia.

The tests check for fetal abnormalities and other conditions – remember that the Foresight programme has been carefully worked out, using all we know about prevention, so that your risks of an abnormal fetus are minimised. If you have been following the programme recommended by Foresight, with your doctor's guidance, you are less likely to be carrying an abnormal baby. This is one of the factors you may wish to bear in mind if you are offered testing facilities.

Tests most commonly used

The tests most commonly used include maternal alpha fetoprotein measures, ultrasound scans, chorion villus biopsy, fetoscopy and amniocentesis.

Maternal alpha fetoprotein – commonly called AFP

This is a blood test done 16 weeks into the pregnancy. (You need to be certain of your dates if it is to be helpful.) Your baby passes to your blood a substance called alpha fetoprotein, the level of which is measured in your blood sample. At 16–19 weeks the level is normally low, although it rises as the pregnancy advances. If the result shows it is higher than expected at this time, then it may indicate that there is an abnormality, such as spina bifida or brain defect. Only about 2 per cent of women have a raised level. In only about 1 in 20 of these are there real problems. In others it may be a multiple pregnancy or the pregnancy may be more advanced than was thought.[3] There could even have been an error at the laboratory. If there is a raised level, you may be offered another test, followed by an ultrasound scan.

However, some research has suggested a failure rate of 20 per cent. In this the AFP level was not raised but subsequently a baby was born with a neural tube defect.[4] It is also known for normal babies to have been born to mothers with high AFP levels.[5]

Ultrasound scanning

Ultrasound scanning, commonly called the 'Scan', is a technique in which ultrasonic waves are beamed into the uterus and bounce off the fetus and the placenta. Using a video screen to record the sound, a skilled operator can see the developing fetus, and interpret the picture. For those who are not skilled, it is very blurred but most women are quite thrilled to see even a blurred image. Some obstetricians believe that seeing the fetus can help the bonding between mother and baby even before birth, though this can also happen in other ways. (See Chapter 5 – manganese and zinc.)

Scans can be used to check the age of the baby, if they are done early in the pregnancy. They also show the baby's growth, and can be used to monitor for growth retardation. They pick up abnormalities, such as neural tube defects, or kidney conditions. They show the position and condition of the placenta. They can ascertain the exact position of the fetus during amniocentesis and thus reduce the risk of this test considerably. They will reveal if there is more than one fetus, as well as any growths in the mother which can impede delivery.

With so many uses, it is not surprising that they are widely performed, and that their frequency of use is increasing. Many women are offered more than one scan during their pregnancy, though not all doctors agree with this. Ultrasound waves are a form of non-ionising radiation and although they are said to be safe, especially now that very weak waves are used, this has yet to be proven. The American College of Radiology has spoken out against routine use in its 'Commission on Ultrasound'.[6] The US government agency, the National Center for Devices and Radiological Health of the Food and Drug Administration published a report saying, 'We can be reasonably certain that acute, dramatic effects are not likely ...But studies have not been made to detect less obvious effects, and the question of subtle, long-term or cumulative effects remains unanswered. The potential for acute adverse effects has not been systematically explored, and the potential for delayed effects has been virtually ignored.'[7]

The two main hazards of ultrasound are heat and cavitation. It is thought that the rises in temperature are too small to cause damage as little heat is produced in pulsed waves of ultrasound. Cavitation, in which air bubbles expand and contract in response to the sound waves, may occur in humans, producing, among other effects, the release of free radicals.[8] Doris Haire, the President of the American Foundation for Maternal and Child Health, at a symposium in 1983, quoted studies suggesting premature ovulation after ovarian ultrasound, damage to maternal blood cells, a higher incidence of leukemia in exposed children, and lower birth weight.[9] However, the results of some of the studies are not significant and there are problems with the research methods. Another researcher has suggested that 'animal studies have been reported to reveal delayed neuro-muscular development, altered emotional behaviour, EEG changes, anomalies and decreased survival'.[10]

The Consumers Association has said, 'Women who are offered a routine scan should be informed not only why it is recommended, but also that it is not an essential part of their antenatal care.'[11] This is a position supported by Foresight. The data on risks is limited, but we must remember that 'absence of proof is not proof of absence!'

Chorion villus biopsy
This test is done between 8 and 12 weeks of pregnancy. It involves taking a small tissue sample from where the embryo joins the placenta, the chorion villi, either by a transcervical biopsy (through the vagina) or by a transabdominal biopsy (through the walls of the stomach). The sample can then be used to check for abnormalities, such as Down's syndrome, sex-linked abnormalities, sickle cell anaemia and muscular dystrophy. The sex can also be determined.

The main advantage quoted of the test is that it can be done in the first three months of pregnancy, allowing time for an early abortion if this is the decision made as a result of the test outcome. However, there are a number of risks. Immediate complications can include perforations of the amniotic sac, severe bleeding (rare), mild to moderate bleeding in under 10 per cent of cases, infection, and foeto-maternal haemorrhage leading to isoimmunisation.[12] There is an increased risk of miscarriage but it is difficult to assess.[13] 2–3 per cent is quoted, but this should not be taken as accurate. Indeed, one study assesses the risk for transcervical biopsy as much higher. London hospital experience suggests a miscarriage rate of over 10 per cent, though the figures in other studies vary between 3 and 30 per cent. From a total of 91 patients tested using the transabdominal route there was only one miscarriage.[14] However, there is no mention in the study of the health of the neonate, nor of subsequent development. Very serious consideration should be given to the risk of miscarriage in women over 40 years of age carrying a much wanted baby as the chances of another conception may be less at this age.

Fetoscopy

This is a method of looking into the womb, used after 15–18 weeks. A very small tube is passed through the amniotic fluid so that the doctor can see the developing fetus direct. He can check for abnormalities such as brain disorders, blood disorders, and cleft palate, and even perform direct therapy to the fetus, such as blood transfusions. However, the test should only be done where there is a high risk to the fetus as it is a dangerous technique for the fetus. The rate of miscarriage is said by one authority to be 3 per cent, though it could be higher.[15] The incidence of other risks is not known but the possibility of infections being introduced by the method cannot be ruled out.

Amniocentesis

This test checks the amniotic fluid, in which the baby floats. A long hollow needle is inserted through the stomach wall into the fluid and a sample is drawn up. It should always be performed in conjunction with an ultrasound scan to ensure that the needle is in the right place to minimise the risks of piercing the fetus. The fluid contains cells from the baby which can be used to test for many conditions, including spina bifida, Down's syndrome and some types of muscular dystrophy.

It is not a routine test and will generally only be offered where there is a high risk to the fetus. Such cases would include situations where the mother may be the carrier of a genetically linked disorder such as haemophilia or muscular dystrophy, or be at risk of a baby with a chromosomal abnormality, such as Down's syndrome. If her AFP level is high or if she will need a caesarian section it may be done.

Amniocentesis is normally performed in or after the 16th week of pregnancy, and since the results can take from three to five weeks to come through, the pregnancy may be well advanced by the time a decision about an abortion can be made. If such a choice has to be considered, one must weigh it against the fact that late abortion is very distressing, both physically and psychologically, for all concerned.

It is difficult to assess the risks of amniocentesis, though they are often quoted as about 1.5 per cent risk of miscarriage. (This is in addition to the usual risk of miscarriage.) The studies that have been done are mostly flawed in some way when one tries to assess the results statistically, as there are many factors which can also cause fetal loss, which cannot be taken into account when doing the research but which may raise the risk figures. However, in their excellent review of all the studies done up to 1986, Ager and Oliver say that, overall, the results indicate that there is a *real* risk to the fetus.[16] They report on research done in Denmark which they claim is the best study undertaken to date. In this, the rate of spontaneous abortion was significantly higher than in the control group, being 1.7 per cent to 0.7 per cent.[17]

It is sometimes claimed that the adverse effects to the woman appear to be very small,[18] though this is hard to understand, since any risks to the fetus must affect the woman. These risks include fetal death, miscarriage, vaginal bleeding followed by miscarriage, and stillbirth, all of which affect the woman. The risks seem to be increased if the obstetrician is not skilled. This is not surprising when one considers that the two main events which cause fetal death are needle damage and the introduction of infection.[19]

Other risks listed by the Medical Research Council report included an increased incidence of neonatal respiratory distress in about 3 per cent of offspring and an increased number of congenital dislocations of the hip and talipes in 2.4 per cent of offspring.[20]

In summary, one should note that 'In evaluating the benefits of amniocentesis it should not be forgotten that the indications are relative and the risks not insignificant'.[21]

X-rays (see Chapter 10)
It would be rare for you to be offered an X-ray for diagnostic or screening purposes during your pregnancy, as it can be very harmful to the fetus. This is why you should always let your doctor or dentist know you are pregnant. If anyone wants to X-ray you, you should be quite certain that it is essential before you consent.

Conclusion
Whatever the claims made by the medical profession about the safety of prenatal screening tests, the research to date is only certain about two things: there are risks and these risks have yet to be properly assessed.

Checklist

In considering the decision about testing, you should ask a number of questions:
1. Would you have an abortion if something was wrong?
2. Are you satisfied with the reasons put forward for the test?

3. What experience has the person who is doing the test?
4. Have you suffered any illness in the first 11 weeks of the pregnancy?
5. Can you cope with the stress of waiting for the results?

Did your preconception care include the following?
6. Was rubella immunity checked prior to your pregnancy?
7. Did you start the pregnancy, to the best of your knowledge, free from high levels of toxic metals?
8. Were you checked for genito-urinary infections, including sexually transmitted ones, and did you have any necessary treatment before conception?
9. Did you have your mineral levels checked?
10. Did you smoke, drink or take drugs during the first 11 weeks of pregnancy?

CHAPTER 15

Postscript

HOW WE CAN ALL HELP EACH OTHER TO HELP THE CHILDREN OF TOMORROW.

The time has come to try and draw our conclusions from the preceding chapters. Each of you will have picked up the book with a different set of experiences, hopes and beliefs, and each of you will put it down with a different mixture of feelings about what can be done for future generations. We hope that you feel that preconceptual care has a part to play. Since the first day dawned it has been the prerogative of parents to instigate necessary change to ensure their children's welfare. It has been almost entirely due to this that the human race has continued to advance. So today, as the active grass roots, how can we most effectively *sprout* to make a 'green and pleasant land' for those to come?

At a very uncomplicated personal level, here are some suggestions and you can doubtless add to them.

- Help the Foresight organisation to continue to research and promote preconceptual care until it is available for one and all, by joining us.
- Help the preconception scene by putting into practice the principles as outlined in this book in the way that best suits your family.
- Help the food scene by buying only fresh 'living' food whenever possible, leaving the white flour, sugar and chemicals on the shelf. Buy flour that is whole and organic. If your supermarket does not yet stock organic meat, fruit and vegetables, tell the manager you would like to be able to buy them. Also, do support your local organic farms and organic pick your own: the more they flourish, the more they can help us.
- Help the Natural Family Planning scene by introducing people to the idea of natural family planning (plus or minus barriers for fertile days). If you have any spare time, perhaps you could learn to teach it? The Natural Family Planning Centres run courses to instruct teachers, and they do need more teachers. (See Appendix One for addresses.)
- Help fight toxic metal by buying lead-free petrol. Many cars run

POSTSCRIPT

on it already: others could be adapted for minimal cost. The AA supplies information on this for members, and your local dealer can also advise you.
- Get drinking water checked for lead, copper, cadmium and aluminium. If any one of these is above the EEC recommended level make a complaint to the Environmental Health Officer. It is also worth telling your Community Health Council and your GP for their information since other houses locally are likely to be the same. Grants are available for house owners to replace obsolete lead plumbing, although this is not widely publicised. If you do this the water authority is obliged to replace the connecting pipe between the mains and the property boundary. This is worth doing both for the benefit of your own family and for those who own the house after you.
- Help to spur the research into safer dental amalgams. Ask about alternatives to mercury-containing amalgams if you need dental repair. New materials are being developed.
- Help the safer kitchenware scene: avoid buying aluminium cookware, kettles, teapots and foil.
- Help the spread of information. If they do not already do so, suggest to your local library, bookshop and/or health store they stock books on preconceptual care, natural family planning, natural childbirth, breastfeeding, nutrition, wholefood cooking, organic growing, allergic illness and natural therapies. When they do, let your GP, midwife and health visitor know they are there.
- Encourage these shops to display information on the whereabouts of local organic growers and Natural Family Planning teachers – the organisations could supply their own posters!
- Suggest local groups give talks on the above subjects. There are many good speakers available. (See Appendix One for addresses.)

So what of the future? The research quoted, coupled with the Foresight findings, leads us to believe that if environmental reforms were achieved and if preconceptual education and preparation were available for all, we could be living in a very different world in the year 2,000.

I think it is realistic to assume we could have hugely reduced rates of sterility, infertility, miscarriage, baby death, and malformed, ill or mentally afflicted babies. I think it is also quite logical to believe we would live in a world where the figures for degenerative disease, 'psychosomatic' illness (usually linked with deficiency and allergy) and psychosis would plummet. Many studies, and our own experience, lead us to be hopeful that dyslexia, hyperactivity and other learning and behaviour problems might become things of the past.

Will tomorrow's child be born sickly and fretful, small, possibly malformed or 'minimally' brain damaged by pollutants, infection and inadequate nourishment? Will he or she be dogged by damaging toxins and allergic illness, with all the emotional and mental consequences? Will he or she be 'creeping like snail unwillingly to school', where hyperactivity, dyslexia and inability to concentrate will make every hour a burden – for both child and teachers? Will the disappointment of poor results, disapprobation and fatigue drive him or her to truancy, alcohol, drugs and bitter relationships? Are these the seeds of squalor, vice, addiction and criminal activity?

Or can we build for tomorrow's child a future free from yesterday's mistakes?

Can he or she be born well nourished and in very good order to rejoicing parents? Can he or she look forward to abundant love and breastmilk and a future full of the joys of comfortably rude health? Natural feeding means less crying, sounder sleep, eventual slow, gentle weaning, less likelihood of allergies and better assimilation of food.

A well-nourished brain means a bright, curious, conversational little child who finds life a rewarding experience, and sees 'grownups' as quite friendly and reasonable! There will be disagreements, of course, with small people who lack experience, and there will be escapades! However, relationships and learning hold great potential when the developing brain is free from biochemical aberration.

Dare we dream that with this help and information coupled with a little extra effort to prepare for a child's welcome, we can get it RIGHT and can give birth to tomorrow's child undamaged, naturally healthy, naturally able, naturally loving?

Dare we dream that maybe he or she will have the guts, the purpose, the integrity, the understanding and the ability NOT to destroy this green and pleasant planet we are striving to preserve for our children? Dare we dream that he or she may nurture and pass on this fertile, living, glorious spinning miracle to all our grandchildren?

For tomorrow's child is everyman's eternity.

Glossary

Abortifacient – causing abortion.
AID – artificial insemination by donor.
Anorexia – lack or loss of appetite, resulting in an inability to eat.
Ataxia – an inability to control voluntary muscle movements.
Atherosclerosis – fatty degeneration and hardening of the arteries.
Atrophy – wasting away, either from lack of use or malnutrition.
Bradycardia – abnormally slow but regular heartbeat.
Bronchoconstriction – tightening of the bronchial tubes.
Candida albicans – the fungus which causes thrush. It occurs naturally in the body but may multiply out of control and cause a condition called candidiasis.
Carcinogen – a substance which causes cancer.
Cervicitis – inflammation of the cervix.
Chelate – pronounced 'Kee-late' – a substance which inactivates heavy metals and enables the body to be cleansed of them.
Chloroprene – a colourless liquid used in the manufacture of neoprene rubber.
Chorioamniocentesis – a test performed at 11 weeks pregnancy to detect Down's syndrome.
Coeliac disease – a condition in which the protein gluten, found in wheat and some other grains, is not tolerated by the body.
Colposcope – an instrument which enables a more detailed gynaecological examination to be made.
DNA – deoxyribose nucleic acid – the complex chemical found in every cell which contains the genetic information.
Dolomite – a natural mineral supplement of calcium and magnesium.
Dysplasia – a metabolic defect in the calcification of the bone.
Eclampsia – a condition in pregnancy in which there are convulsions.
Ectopic pregnancy – pregnancy occurring outside the womb.
Encephalopathy – a disease of the brain.
Endometriosis – a condition in which the type of tissue which lines the womb grows outside the womb.
Exencephaly – a congenital defect in which the brain is completely exposed or protrudes through a defect in the skull.
Formaldehyde – toxic gas used to make wet-strength resins and in some house insulation.
Hydrocephalus – a condition in which fluid accumulates in the skull.
Hyperemesis – excessive sickness.
In utero – in the womb.
In vitro fertilisation – IVF – the fertilisation of the egg in a test-tube.
Intracranial calcification – the deposition of calcium inside the skull.
Isoimmunisation – sensitisation of the mother to her baby's blood.

Klinefelter's syndrome – a rare condition in which the male genitalia are congenitally deformed.
Lactation – the time or process of suckling young.
Libido – sexual desire or impulse.
Macrocephaly – having an excessively large head.
Male accessory (sex) organs – gonads, prostate, seminal vesicles, bulbourethral glands and ampulla of the ductus deferens – which produce secretory products that protect and affect the viability and fertilising potential of the sperm.
Microcephaly – having an abnormally small head.
Microphthalmia – having abnormally small eyes.
Mutagen – a substance which causes changes in the cells of the body.
Myelin – the substance which forms a sheath round the nerve.
Necrosis – death of the tissue.
Neonate – the child in the first month of life (after birth).
Neural tube defects – NTD – defects of the nervous system, such as spina bifida.
Neuritis – inflammation of the nerve or nerves.
Neurotoxicity – poisonous effect on nerves and nerve cells.
Oedema – swelling.
Oestrogen – a female sex hormone.
Organochlorines – organic compounds containing chlorine, including chloroform, DDT and other pesticides.
Osteomalacia – softening of the bones.
Osteoporosis – a condition in which the bones become very brittle.
Otitis media – inflammation of the middle ear.
Polychlorinated biphenyls – PCBs – toxic chemicals used in electrical components.
Postpartum depression – postnatal depression – depression occurring after childbirth.
Pre-eclamptic toxemia – a condition with high blood pressure which may lead to eclampsia.
Proctitis – inflammation of the rectum.
Progesterone – female sex hormone.
Progestogen – substance like progesterone, which is found in contraceptive pills.
Psychomotor retardation – delay in acquiring skills which involve both mental and muscular activity, such as sitting, walking, grasping and talking.
Reactive hypoglycaemia – also called hypoglycaemia and functional hypoglycaemia – deficiency of sugar in the blood.
Rhinitis – inflammation of the mucous membranes in the nose.
Spermatozoa – the male reproductive cells.
Talipes – clubfoot.
Teratogen – a substance which harms the fetus.
Tonic/clonic convulsions – a grand mal seizure: alternating tonic (rigid muscles) and clonic (jerking of muscles) phases.
Vulvitis – inflammation of the vulva – the external sex organs of the female.

Appendix One

LIST OF USEFUL ADDRESSES

Action Against Allergy
43 The Downs
Wimbledon
London SW20
Tel 01-947 5082

Active Birth Movement
The Active Birth Centre
Dartmouth Park Road
London NW5

AIMS
Association for the Improvement of Maternity Services
40 Kingswood Avenue
London NW6

ARM
Association of Radical Midwives
62 Greetby Hill
Ormskirk
Lancs L39 2DT

Association for Breastfeeding Mothers
Sydenham Green Health Centre
26 Holmshaw Road
Sydenham
London SE26 4TH

The Billings Method
12 Eastwood
Three Bridges Road
Crawley
West Sussex

Biodynamic Agricultural Association
Broome Farm
Clent
Stourbridge
Worcestershire

Biolab
The Stone House
9 Weymouth Street
London W1

Biosocial Publications
126 High Road
East Finchley
London N2 9ED

Biosocial Therapy Association
115 Hampstead Way
Hampstead Garden Suburb
London NW11 7JN

Brita Water Filters
The Butt Centre
Reading
Berks

British Homeopathic Association
27a Devonshire Street
London W1

British Society for Nutritional Medicine
PO Box 3AP
London W1A 3AP

The Cantassium Company
Larkhall Laboratories
225 Putney Bridge Road
London SW15 2PY

Compassion in World Farming
Lyndham House
Greatham
Petersfield
Hampshire

Environmental Medicine Foundation
6 Jervis Court
Princes Street
London W1R 7RE

FACT (Food Additives Campaign Team)
25 Horsell Road
London N5 1XL

Farm and Food Society
4 Willifield Way
London NW11

Food Allergy Association
9 Mill Lane
Shoreham by Sea
West Sussex

Foodwatch
Butts Pond Industrial Estate
Sturminster Newton
Dorset
DT10 1AZ

Foresight
The Old Vicarage
Church Lane
Witley
Godalming
Surrey GU8 5PN

Friends of the Earth
26–28 Underwood Street
London N1 7JQ

The Good Gardeners' Association
Arkley Manor
Rowley Lane
Arkley
Barnet
Herts EN5 3HS

Health Education Authority
76 New Oxford Street
London WC1

Henry Doubleday Research Association
Ryton-on-Dunsmore
Coventry
Warwickshire CV8 3LG

Hyperactive Children's Support Group
71 Whyke Lane
Chichester
Sussex

La Leche League
Spencer Lester
30 Whimbrel Way
Banbury
Oxon OX16 9YN

London Food Commission
PO Box 291
London N5 1DU

Maternity Alliance
59–61 Camden High Street
London NW1 7JL

The Mayrei Water Filter
La Source de Vie
PO Box 66
Chichester
Sussex

The McCarrison Society
24 Paddington Street
London W1M 4DR

National Centre for Alternative Technology
Llwyngwern Quarry
Machynlleth
Powys

National Childbirth Trust
Alexandra House
Oldham Terrace
Acton
London W3 6NH

Natural Family Planning Centre
Birmingham Maternity Hospital
Queen Elizabeth Medical Centre
Edgbaston
Birmingham B15 2TG
Tel 021-472 1377 Ext 285

Also:

Mrs Colleen Norman
218 Heathwood Road
Heath
Cardiff
S. Wales
Welsh NFP office Tel Cardiff 493120 mornings

National Society for Research into Allergy
PO Box 45
Hinckley
Leicestershire LE10 1JY

LIST OF USEFUL ADDRESSES

Organic Food Services
Ashe Churston Ferres
Nr Brixham
Devon

Organic Growers Association
Aeron Park
Llangietho
Dyfed

Pesticide Pressure Group Sufferers
10 Parker Street
Cambridge CB1 1JL

Pill Victims Association
Mrs Judith Challenger
3 Eney Close
Abingdon
Oxford

Schizophrenia Association of Great Britain
Bryn Hyfryd
The Crescent
Bangor
Gwynedd LL57 2AG

Society for Environmental Therapy
Mrs H. Davidson
521 Foxhall Road
Ipswich
Suffolk IP3 8LW

Soil Association
86 Colston Street
Bristol BS1 5BB

Support After Termination For Abnormalities (SAFTA)
29 Soho Square
London W1

Templegarth Trust
82 Tinkly Street
Grimoldby
Louth
Lincs LN11 8TF

The Vegetarian Society
53 Marlowe Road
London W8 6LA

Vitamin Service
Littlewick Road
Lower Knaphill
Woking
Surrey

The Westminster Advisory Centre on Alcoholism
38 Ebury Street
London SW1W 0LU

Wholefood
24 Paddington Street
London W1M 4DR

Working Weekends on Organic Farms (WWOOF)
19 Bradford Road
Lewes
Sussex BN7 1RB

The World Federation of Doctors who respect human life
c/o Dr Peggy Norris
79 St Mary's Road
Huyton
Merseyside L36 5SR

Appendix Two

RECOMMENDED READING LIST

Pregnancy and parenthood
A Child is Born. Lars Neilsson. Faber Paperbacks. 1977.
At Highest Risk. Christopher Norwood. McGraw-Hill. 1980.
Building Better Babies. Daniel Elam. Celestial Arts. 1980.
Guidelines For Future Parents. Foresight. 1985.
The First Nine Months of Life. Geraldine Lux Flanagan. Simon and Schuster. 1962.
The Poisoned Womb. John Elkington. Viking. 1985.
The Prevention of Handicap and the Health of Women. Margaret and Arthur Wynn. Routledge and Kegan Paul. 1979.
The Prevention of Handicap of Perinatal Origin. M. and A. Wynn. Foundation for Education and Research in Child Bearing. 1976.
The Prevention of Preterm Birth. M. and A. Wynn. Foundation for Education and Research in Child Bearing. 1977.
What Every Pregnant Woman Should Know. The Truth about Diets, and Drugs and Pregnancy. G. S. and T. Brewer. Penguin. 1977.

Nutrition
'Effect of Heat Processed Foods on the Dento-facial Structures of Experimental Animals.' F. M. Pottenger. *American Journal of Orthodontics and Oral Surgery*, Vol 32, No 8, Oral Surgery Pages 467–485, August 1946. Reprint available from Wholefood (see addresses).
Mental and Elemental Nutrients. Carl C. Pfeiffer. Keats. 1975.
Nutrition and Health. Sir Robert McCarrison. The McCarrison Society. 1981.
Nutrition and Physical Degeneration. Weston A. Price. Price-Pottenger Nutrition Foundation. 1945.
Nutrition and Vitamin Therapy. Michael Lesser. Bantam. 1980.
Metabolic Toxemia of Late Pregnancy. A Disease of Malnutrition. T. S. Brewer. Keats Publishing. 1982. Conn, USA.
'Physical Degeneration and Allergic Diathesis.' Granville F. Knight. *The Transactions, American Society of Opthalmologic and Otolaryngologic Allergy*. Vol 9, No 1, 1968. Reprint available from Wholefood (see addresses).
Pottenger's Cats: A Study in Nutrition. F. M. Pottenger. Price-Pottenger. Nutrition Foundation. 1983.
Let's Eat Right To Keep Fit. Adelle Davis. Signet Books. 1970.
Raw Energy. Leslie and Susannah Kenton. Century. 1984.
The Food Factor. Barbara Griggs. Penguin. 1988.
Trace Elements in Human and Animal Nutrition. Eric J. Underwood. Academic Press. 1977.
The Healing Nutrients Within. Eric R. Braverman, with Carl Pfeiffer. Keats. 1987.
Total Nutrition During Pregnancy. Betty and Si Kamen. Appleton-Century-Crofts. 1981.
Trace Elements, Hair Analysis and Nutrition. Richard A. Passwater and Elmer Cranton. Keats. 1983.
What we eat today. Michael and Sheilagh Crawford. Neville Spearman. 1972.
Zinc and Other Micro-Nutrients. Carl C. Pfeiffer. Keats. 1978.

RECOMMENDED READING LIST

Cookbooks
The Foresight Wholefood Cookbook. Norman and Ruth Jervis. Aurum Press. 1986.
Growing Up with Good Food. Catherine Lewis. Unwin Paperbacks. 1982.
Good Food Before Birth. Catherine Lewis. Unwin Paperbacks. 1984.

Birth control
The Bitter Pill. Ellen Grant. Corgi. 1985.
The Manual of Natural Family Planning. Anna Flynn and Melissa Brooks. Unwin Paperbacks. 1984.

Environmental factors
Green Britain or Industrial Wasteland. Goldsmith and Hildyard. Polity Press. 1986.
The Circle of Poison – Pesticides and Poison in a Hungry World. Weir and Shapiro. Institute of Food and Development Policy. San Francisco. 1981.
Light, Radiation and You. John Ott. Devin-Adair. 1985.
Daylight Robbery. Damien Downing. Century. 1988.
The Green Consumer Guide. John Elkington and Julia Hailes. Gollancz. 1988.

Food additives
Additives. A Guide for Everyone. Erik Millstone. John Abraham. Penguin. 1988.
Find Out. Foresight. 1986.

Health problems
Allergies: Your Hidden Enemy. Theron Randolph. Turnstone Press. 1981.
Chemicals Victims. Richard MacKarness. Pan. 1980.
Everywoman's Book. Paavo Airola. Health Plus Publishers. 1979.
Nutritional Medicine. Stephen Davies and Alan Stewart. Pan. 1987.
The Allergy Problem: Why People Suffer and What Should Be Done. Vicky Rippere. Thorson. 1983.
The Missing Diagnosis. C. Orion Truss. (On candida) M.D. Inc. 1983.

Gardening
Gardening without Chemicals. Jack Temple. Thorsons. 1986.

Appendix Three

FOOD ALLERGY QUESTIONNAIRE

Questionnaire for detection of food allergy

Name

Date

Tick in appropriate column for past/recent symptoms.
(Recent means within the last year.)

		Past	Recent
Headaches	General		
	Migraine		
Face ache	Like sinusitis		
Torso and limbs	Muscular spasm		
	Weakness		
	Paralysis		
	Numbness		
	Tingling		
	Aching – localised		
	Jigging legs		
	Restless legs		
	Shaking hands		
	Aching all over		
Arthritis	One joint		
	Many joints		
	Swollen joint(s)		
	Deformed joint(s)		
Eating problems	Poor appetite		
	Food addictions (most favourite)		
	Binging sessions		
Irritable bowel syndrome	Abdominal discomfort, pains, cramps		
	Nausea		
	Vomiting		
	Sudden diarrhoea		
	Constipation		
	Lots of mucus in stool		
	Belching, flatulence		
Other gastro-intestinal problems	Ulcerative colitis		
	Crohn's disease		

FOOD ALLERGY QUESTIONNAIRE

		Past	Recent
Urinary problems	Frequency Incontinence Late bedwetting Vaginitis Itching genital and/or rectal area		
Heart	Irregular pulse Palpitations Other?		
Hyperventilation	Fast, panting attacks Repeated sighing Repeated yawning Vertigo		
Angioedema	Swelling lips Swelling around the eyes Puffy face Swelling fingers Swelling ankles Swelling limbs Swelling 'all over' Fluctuating daily weight		
Asthma	Exercise induced Sudden attacks Seasonal During respiratory infections		
Medications	Antihistamines Broncho-dilators Steroids		
Other	Frequent throat clearing Recurrent cough not responding to treatment		
Rhinitis	Frequent runny nose Seasonal runny nose Frequent catarrh Seasonal catarrh Snorting noises Itchy nose Polyps		
Conjunctivitis	Itchy watery eyes Seasonal? Reddened eyes Seasonal?		
Skin problems	Eczema – itchy red patches Urticaria – nettle rash, welts Contact dermatitis – local itchy blisters		

		Past	Recent
Scalp	Dandruff		
Sensitivity	Very oversensitive to touch		
Mouth problems	Scaling cracked lips		
	Mouth ulcers		
	Repeated cold sores		
	Geographic tongue, patchy or spotty		
	Bad breath		
	Itchy skin after some foods		
Otitis	Ear aches, repeated		
	Deafness from fluid in ears		
	Bad dizziness		
Psychological symptoms	Chronic fatigue		
	Dysthymia		
	Agitation, tension, irritability		
	Hyperactivity		
	Anxiety, panic attacks		
	Abrupt mood changes		
	Insomnia		
	Short term memory loss		
	Stupor, 'coma'		
	Petit mal		
	Convulsions or fits, grand mal		
	Violent outbursts, attacks		
	Self mutilation		
	Psychotic behaviour		
	Mania		
	True depression		
	Auditory hallucinations		
	Visual hallucinations		
	Depersonalisation		
	Separate personalities		
	Multiple personalities		
	Schizoid withdrawal		
Medication			
Use of drugs			

FOOD ALLERGY QUESTIONNAIRE

		Past	Recent
Other allergies	Insect stings where reaction is worse than usual		
	Toxaemia		
	Animals		
	Feathers, birds		
	Dust, bedding, dirty houses		
	Paint		
	Drugs and medicines, aspirin		
	Perfume		
	Suspected foods		
	Cigarette smoke		
	Chemicals		
	Traffic fumes		
	Chemicals		
	Other		
Allergic symptoms in family	Mother		
	Father		
	Siblings		
	Grandparents		
	Epilepsy in family?		
	Mental illness in family?		
	Dyslexia in family?		

Other comments

References

Chapter 3

1. Judges, 13, 3–4
2. Price, Weston A., *Nutrition and Physical Degeneration*. La Mesa, CA, Price-Pottenger Foundation, 1945, 397
3. Hoffer, A., 'Orthomolecular Nutrition at the Zoo.' *Orthomolecular Psychiatry*, 1983, 12(2), 116–128
4. Sutherland, Hamish, *Lancet*, 1982, 1
5. Black, Sir Douglas, et al., *Inequalities in Health: the Black Report*, Harmondsworth, Penguin, 1982
6. OPCS Monitor, Reference DH3 84/2, Issued 1 May 1984
7. WHO, World Health Statistics, 1976–1985, Geneva, WHO
8. WHO, World Health Statistics, 1986, Geneva, WHO
9. Lambert, P., 'Perinatal Mortality: Social and Environmental Factors.' In: *Population Trends 4*, London, HMSO, Summer 1976, 4–8
10. See WHO, World Health Statistics, as in ref 7 above
11. OPCS Monitor, Reference MB3 87/1, Issued 22 September 1987, 4
12. Andrews, Lori B., *New Conceptions*, New York, St Martin's Press, 1984, 2
13. Dougherty, Ralph. In: *Anon. Unplugging the Gene Pool*, Outside, September 1980, 13
14. Magenis, P.E., et al., 'Parental origin of the extra chromosome in down's syndrome', *Human Genetics*, 1977, 37, 7–16
15. West, Christine P., 'Age and Infertility', *British Medical Journal*, 1987, 294, 853
16. Varma, T.R., 'Infertility', *British Medical Journal*, 1987, 294, 887–890
17. Hull, Michael, *The Agony and the Ecstasy*, Channel 4 TV, 14 April 1988
18. Prentice, Thomson, 'Anguish of the Sterile Husbands,' *The Times*, 20 April 1988, 3
19. Huisjes, H.J., 'Spontaneous Abortion'. In: *Current Reviews in Obstetrics and Gynecology*, Edinburgh, Churchill Livingstone, 1984
20. Bell, L.T., et al., 'Chromosomal abnormalities in maternal and fetal tissues of magnesium and zinc in deficient rats', *Teratology*, 1975, 12, 221–226
21. Annis, Linda Ferrill, *The Child Before Birth*, London and Ithaca, Cornell University Press, 1978, 133
22. Ward, N.I., et al., 'Placental Element Levels In Relation To Fetal Development for Obstetrically "Normal" Births: A Study Of 37 Elements. Evidence For Effects Of Cadmium, Lead, And Zinc On Fetal Growth, And Smoking As A Source Of Cadmium.' *Int J Biosocial Res*, 1987, 9(1), 63–81
23. Grant, Ellen, *The Bitter Pill*, London, Corgi, 1985, 162
24. Annis, Linda Ferrill, *op cit.*, 135
25. *Ibid*, 136–137
26. Kamen, Betty and Si, *The Kamen Plan For Total Nutrition During Pregnancy*, New York, Appleton-Century-Crofts, 1981, 24–30. This summarises a number of studies.
27. Avery, Mary Ellen, Litwack, Georgia, *Born Early. The Story of a Premature Baby*, Boston, Little Brown and Company, 1983, 19
28. Nance, Sherri, *Premature Babies*, Arbour House, 1982
29. Naeye, R.L., Peters, E.D., 'Work during pregnancy: effects on the fetus.' *Pediatrics*, 1982, 69, 724–727
30. Douglas, Charles P., 'Low birthweight – preterm and small'. In: eds Chamberlain, Geoffrey, *Contemporary Obstetrics*, London, Butterworths, 1984, 218–226
31. Annis, Linda Ferrill, *op cit.*, 135
32. Churchill, John A., et al., 'Birth Weight and Intelligence,' *Obstet Gynecol*, 1966, 28, 425–429
33. Holiverda-Kuipers, J., 'The cognitive development of low birthweight children,' *J Child Psychology and Psychiat*, 1987, 28, 321–328
34. Spiers, P.S., 'Does Growth Retardation Predispose the Fetus to Congenital Malformations?', *Lancet*, 1982, i, 312–314
35. Annis, Linda Ferrill, *op cit.*, 139
36. Spyker, Joan M., 'Occupational Hazards and the Pregnant Worker,' *Behavioural Toxicology Overview*, 470

Chapter 4

1. Davies, Stephen, 'Preconceptual care', *Pulse*, 16 June 1984
2. Lodge Rees, E., 'The concept of preconceptual care', *Intern J. Environmental Studies*, 1981, 17, 37–42
3. Wynn, Arthur and Margaret, 'Prevention of Handicap of Early Pregnancy Origin'. Today – Building Tomorrow: International Conference on Physical Disabilities, Montreal, 4–6 June 1986
4. *Ibid*
5. *Ibid*
6. Reading, Chris and Meilon, Ross, *Relatively Speaking*, Sydney, Fontana, 1984
7. Barnes, Broda O., *Hypothyroidism: The Unsuspected Illness*, London and New York, Harper and Row, 1976
8. Consumers Association
9. 'Face the Facts', BBC Radio 4, 19 January 1988
10. Laker, Martin, 'On determining trace element levels in man: the uses of blood and hair', *Lancet*, 1982, ii, 260–262
11. Klevay, Leslie M., 'Hair as a Biopsy Material. Progress and Prospects', *Arch Intern Med*, 1978, 138, 1127–1128
12. Maugh, Thomas H. II, 'Hair: A Diagnostic Tool to Complement Blood Serum and Urine', *Science*, 1978, 202, 1271–1273
13. Gordon, Garry F., 'Hair Analysis: Its Current Use and Limitations', *Let's Live*, October 1980, 54–62
14. Gordon, Garry F., 'Hair Analysis: Its Current Use and Limitations. Part II', *Let's Live*, November 1980, 89–94
15. Fletcher, David J., 'Hair Analysis: Proven and problematic applications', *Postgrad Medicine*, 1982, 72(5), 79–88
16. Passwater, Richard A. and Cranton, Elmer M., *Trace Elements, Hair Analysis and Nutrition*, New Canaan, NC, Keats, 1983

REFERENCES

17. Coleman, R.F. et al., 'The trace element content of human head hair in England and Wales and the application to forensic science.' Paper presented by R.F. Coleman at the International Conference on Forensic Activation Analysis in San Diego, 19–22 September 1966
18. Barrett, S., 'Commercial Hair Analysis: Science or Scam?', *J Am Med Assn*, 1985, 25(8), 1041–1045
19. Barrett, S., *op. cit.*
20. Schoenthaler, Stephen J., 'Commercial Hair Analysis: Lack of Reference Norms and High Reliability Within and Between Seven Selected Laboratories for Seventeen Trace Minerals', *Int J Biosocial Res.*, 1986(1), 84–92
21. Editorial, *Lancet*, 9 November 1985
22. Gordon, Garry F., 'Toxic Metals, Health and Hair Analysis'
23. Vitale, Leonard F. et al., 'Blood Lead – An Inadequate Measure of Occupational Exposure', *J Occ Med*, 1975, 17, 102–103
24. Chattopadhyay, Amares, et al., 'Scalp Hair as a Monitor of Community Exposure to Lead', *Arch Envirn Health*, 1977
25. Passwater, Richard A. and Cranton, Elmer M., *op. cit.*, 278
26. *Ibid*, 288
27. *Ibid*, 284
28. Klevay, *op. cit.*, 1127
29. Maugh, *op. cit.*, 1272–1273
30. Gordon, ref 12 above
31. Lesser, Michael, *Nutrition and Vitamin Therapy*, New York, Bantam, 1980
32. Cott, Allan, *Help for Your Learning Disabled Child. The Orthomolecular Treatment*, New York, Times Books, 1985
33. Schauss, Alexander G., *Diet, Crime and Delinquency*, Berkeley, Parker House, 1979
34. Lodge Rees, Elizabeth, 'Prevention versus Problems in Paediatric Practice'. In *The Next Generation*, Anon, Witley, Surrey, Foresight, 1983, 2–12
35. Gordon, ref 12 above
36. Maugh, *op. cit.*, 1272–1273
37. Barnes, Belinda, *A Lay Person's Interpretation*, Witley, Surrey, Foresight, 1987
38. Lodge Rees, Elizabeth, *op. cit.*, 8
39. Price, Weston A., *Nutrition and Physical Degeneration*, La Mesa, CA, Price-Pottenger Foundation, 1945

Chapter 5

1. Williams, Roger J., *Nutrition Against Disease*, New York, Bantam, 1973, 53
2. Rosso, P., Lederman, S.A., 'Nutrition in Pregnancy', In *Proceedings of the 10th study group of the Royal College of Obstetricians and Gynaecologists*, Ed. Campbell, D.M., Gillmer, M.D.G., September 1982, 115–130
3. Williams, Roger J., *op. cit.*, 53–54
4. Health Education Council. A discussion paper on proposals for nutritional guidelines for health education in Britain. Prepared for the National Advisory Committee on Nutrition Education by an ad hoc working party under the Chairmanship of Professor W.P.T. James. NACNE, September 1983
5. DHSS-COMA, *Diet and cardiovascular disease*, London, HMSO 1984
6. Report of the Board of Science and Education, *Diet, Nutrition and Health*, British Medical Association, March 1986
7. The Health Education Council (now the Health Education Authority) has issued many booklets, as well as the NACNE report (ref 4 above). See, for example, *Beating Heart Disease*, undated
8. Price, Weston A., *Nutrition and Physical Degeneration*, La Mesa, Price-Pottenger Nutrition Foundation, 1945
9. Pottenger, F.M. Jnr., *Pottenger's Cats*, La Mesa, CA, Price-Pottenger Nutrition Foundation 1983
10. McCarrison, Sir Robert, *Nutrition and Health*, London, McCarrison Society 1984
11. Williams, Roger J., *Biochemical individuality: the basis for the genetotrophic concept*, New York, Wiley 1956
12. Pfeiffer, Carl C., *Zinc and Other Micronutrients*, New Canaan, Keats, 1978
13. Lesser, Michael, *Nutrition and Vitamin Therapy*, New York, Bantam, 1980
14. Hawkins, David, Pauling, Linus, *Orthomolecular Psychiatry, Treatment of Schizophrenia*, San Francisco, CA, W.H. Freeman and Company 1973
15. Wynn, Arthur and Margaret, 'Prevention of Handicap of Early Pregnancy Origin', Today – Building Tomorrow: International Conference on Physical Disabilities, Montreal, 4 to 6 June 1986. First Session
16. Antonov, A.N., 'Children Born during the Siege of Leningrad in 1942', *J Pediatr*, 1947, 30, 250–259
17. Smith, G.A., 'Effects of maternal undernutrition upon the newborn infant in Holland' (1944–1945), *J Pediatr*, 1947, 30, 250–259
18. Pickard, Barbara, *Guidelines for Future Parents*, Witley, Foresight, 1986, 41
19. Kamen, Betty and Si, *The Kamen Plan for Total Nutrition During Pregnancy*, New York, Appleton-Century-Crofts 1981, 21–30. This gives a good overview of weight gain during pregnancy
20. Montagu, Ashley, *Life Before Birth*, New York, New American Library 1961, 23
21. Reusens, B. et al., 'Controlling Factors of Fetal Nutrition'. In eds: Sutherland, H.W., Stowers, J.M., *Carbohydrate Metabolism in Pregnancy*, New York, Springer-Verlag, 1979, 209
22. Laurence, K.M. et al., 'Increased risk of recurrence of neural tube defects to mothers on poor diets and the possible benefits of dietary counselling', *British Medical Journal*, 1980, 281, 1509–1511
23. Mortimer, G. Rosen, *In The Beginning: Your Baby's Brain Before Birth*, New York, New American Library 1975, 25
24. Cannon, Geoffrey, 'Why Hampstead Babies are 2lbs Heavier', *The Sunday Times*, 28 March 1983
25. Ebrahim, G.J., 'The Problems of Undernutrition'. In Jarrett, R.J. ed., *Nutrition and Disease*, Baltimore, University Park Press, 1979, 29
26. Rush, David et al., 'Diet in Pregnancy: A Randomised Controlled Trial of Nutritional Supplements', *Birth Defects Original Article Series*, Vol 16, No 3, New York, Alan R. Liss Inc, 1980, 114
27. Jervis, Ruth and Norman, *The Foresight Wholefood Cookbook*, London, Roberts Publications 1984
28. Erdmann, Robert, Meiron Jones, *The Amino Revolution*, London, Century Paperbacks 1987, 82
29. Erdmann, Robert, *op. cit.*, 83–84
30. Jervis, Ruth and Norman, *op. cit.*
31. Moore Lappe, Francis, *Diet for a Small Planet*, New York, Ballantine 1975
32. Jervis, Ruth and Norman, *op. cit.*
33. Smyth, Angela, 'Trouble on Tap', *Here's Health*, May 1988, 58–61
34. Mercier, Chas, 'Diet as a Factor in the Causation of Mental Disease', *Lancet*, 1916, i, 561
35. Hurley, Lucille, *Developmental Nutrition*, Englewood Cliffs, NJ, Prentice-Hall, 1980
36. Jennings, I.W., *Vitamins in Endocrine Metabolism*, London, Heinemann 1970, 130–

37. Harrell, Ruth F. et al., 'The Influence of Vitamin Supplementation of the Diets of Pregnant and Lactating Women on the Intelligence of Their Offspring', *Metabolism*, 1956, 5, 555–562
38. Peer, L.A. et al., 'Effect of vitamins on human teratology', *Plast Reconst Surg*, 1964, 34, 358
39. Picciano, Mary Frances, 'Nutrient Needs of Infants', *Nut Today*, Feb 8–13, 1987
40. Baird Cousins, 'Effects of Undernutrition on Central Nervous System Function', *Nutr Reviews*, 1965, 23, 65–68
41. Smith, J.C. et al., 'Alterations in vitamin A metabolism during zinc deficiency and food and growth restriction', *J Nut*, 1976, 106, 569–574
42. Smith, J.C. et al., 'Zinc: a trace element essential in vitamin A metabolism', *Science*, 1973, 181, 954–955
43. Marks, John, *A Guide to the Vitamins*, Lancaster, Medical and Technical Publishing Co Ltd. 1979, 46
44. Hodges, Robert E., Adelman, Raymond D., *Nutrition in Medical Practice*, Philadelphia, W.B. Saunders, 1980, 43
45. Lesser, Michael, *op. cit.*, 92
46. Robson, John, R.K., *Malnutrition: its causation and control*, New York, Gordon and Breach, 1972, 401
47. Hale, F., 'Pigs born without eye balls', *J Hered*, 1935, 24, 105–106
48. Jennings, I.W., *op. cit.*, 43
49. Price, Weston A., *op. cit.*, 333
50. Jennings, I.W., *op. cit.*, 130
51. Jennings, I.W., *op. cit.*, 43
52. Gal, Isobel et al., Vitamin A in relation to human congenital malformations, 149
53. Davis, Adelle, *Let's Eat Right to Keep Fit*, New York, New American Library, 1954, 58
54. Jennings, I.W., *op. cit.*, 131
55. Nutrition Search Inc., *Nutrition Almanac*, New York, McGraw-Hill Book Company, 1979, 94
56. Marks, John, *op. cit.*, 54
57. Lesser, Michael, *op. cit.*, 95
58. Davis, Adelle, *op. cit.*, 143
59. *Ibid*, 143–144
60. *Ibid*, 141
61. Marks, John, *op. cit.*, 58
62. Nutrition Search Inc., *op. cit.*, 96
63. Davis, Adelle, *op. cit.*, 140–141
64. *Ibid*, 154
65. Nutrition Search Inc., *op. cit.*, 53
66. Davis, Adelle, *op. cit.*, 159
67. *Tomorrow's World*, BBC 1, 12 November 1987
68. Davis, Adelle, *op. cit.*, 152–153
69. Williams, Roger J., 1971, *op. cit.*, 253–256
70. Marks, John, *op. cit.*, 63
71. Jennings, I.W., *op. cit.*, 134
72. Davis, Adelle, *op. cit.*, 148
73. *Ibid*, 154
74. Nutrition Search Inc., *op. cit.*, 96
75. *Ibid*, 55
76. Horrobin, David F., 'The Importance of Gamma-Linolenic Acid and Prostaglandin E1 in Human Nutrition and Medicine', *J Holistic Med*, 1981, 3(2), 118–139
77. Graham, Judy, *Evening Primrose Oil*, Wellingborough, Thorsons 1984, 34
78. Horrobin, David. In: Kamen, Betty and Si, *op. cit.*, 186
79. Jennings, I.W., *op. cit.*, 111–112
80. Horrobin, David, 1981, *op. cit.*
81. Colquhoun, Irene, Barnes, Belinda, *The Hyperactive Child. What the Family Can Do*, Wellingborough, Thorsons 1984
82. Nutrition Search Inc., *op. cit.*, 96
83. Marks, John, *op. cit.*, 71
84. Pfeiffer, Carl C., *Mental and Elemental Nutrients*, New Canaan, Connecticut, Keats, 1975, 169–170
85. Jennings, I.W., *op. cit.*, 58
86. Pfeiffer, Carl C., 1975, *op. cit.*, 178
87. Nutrition Search Inc., *op. cit.*, 94
88. *Ibid*, 23
89. Marks, John, *op. cit.*, 79
90. Jennings, I.W., *op. cit.*, 132
91. Hurley, Lucille S., *Developmental Nutrition*, Englewood Cliffs, NJ, Prentice-Hall 1980, 150
92. Pfeiffer, Carl C., 1975, *op. cit.*, 173
93. Marks, John, *op. cit.*, 80
94. Nutrition Search Inc., *op. cit.*, 94
95. Pfeiffer, Carl C., 1975, *op. cit.*, 179
96. Marks, John, *op. cit.*, 89
97. Nutrition Search Inc., *op. cit.*, 24
98. Marks, John, *op. cit.*, 91
99. Jennings, I.W., *op. cit.*, 131–132
100. Hodges, Robert E., Adelman, Raymond D., 'Nutrition in Medical Practice', Philadelphia, W.B. Saunders 1980, 43
101. Robertson, W.F., 'Thalidomide (Distaval) and Vitamin B Deficiency', *British Medical Journal*, 1962, 1, 792
102. Nutrition Search Inc., *op. cit.*, 94
103. Pfeiffer, Carl C., 1975, *op. cit.*, 119–120
104. Nutrition Search Inc., *op. cit.*, 38
105. Marks, John, *op. cit.*, 109
106. Pfeiffer, Carl C., 1975, 120
107. Davis, Adelle, *op. cit.*, 86–87
108. Jennings, I.W., *op. cit.*, 132
109. Nutrition Search Inc., *op. cit.*, 95
110. *Ibid*, 41
111. Davis, Adelle, *op. cit.*, 79–80
112. Jennings, I.W., *op. cit.*, 133
113. Marks, John, *op. cit.*, 129
114. Williams, Roger J., 1973, *op. cit.*, 57
115. Davis, Adelle, *op. cit.*, 70–76
116. Nutrition Search Inc., *op. cit.*, 96
117. *Ibid*, 25
118. Williams, Roger J., 1973, *op. cit.*, 81
119. *Ibid*, 160
120. Pfeiffer, Carl C., *op. cit.*, 146
121. *Ibid*, 151
122. Williams, Roger J., 1973, *op. cit.*, 81
123. Anon, 'Tie Deficiency in Vitamin B6 to Low Agpar', *Medical Tribune*, 2 April 1980, 27
124. Davis, Adelle, *op. cit.*, 83
125. Nutrition Search Inc., *op. cit.*, 94
126. *Ibid*, 37
127. Pfeiffer, Carl C., *op. cit.*, 183
128. Nutrition Search Inc., *op. cit.*, 96
129. *Ibid*, 30
130. Chaitow, Leon, *Candida Albicans. Could Yeast be Your Problem?*, Thorsons, 1984
131. Pfeiffer, Carl C., *op. cit.*, 182
132. Williams, Roger J., 1973, *op. cit.*, 161
133. Davis, Adelle, *op. cit.*, 69
134. Jennings, I.W., *op. cit.*, 132
135. Nutrition Search Inc., *op. cit.*, 95
136. *Ibid*, 33
137. Davis, Adelle, *op. cit.*, 71–73
138. Nutrition Search Inc., *op. cit.*, 95
139. *Ibid*, 31
140. Davis, Adelle, *op. cit.*, 73–76
141. Marks, John, *op. cit.*, 146
142. Williams, Roger J., 1973, *op. cit.*, 186
143. Marks, John, *op. cit.*, 146
144. Nutrition Search Inc., *op. cit.*, 95
145. *Ibid*, 27
146. Pfeiffer, Carl C., *op. cit.*, 157
147. Douglass, John. In: Kamen, Betty and Si, *The Kamen Plan for Total Nutrition During Pregnancy*, New York, Appleton-Century-Crofts 1981, 36
148. Pfeiffer, Carl C., *op. cit.*, 158–160
149. Davis, Adelle, *op. cit.*, 77
150. Marks, John, *op. cit.*, 122
151. *Ibid*, 121
152. Nutrition Search Inc., *op. cit.*, 95
153. *Ibid*, 32
154. Lesser, Michael, *op. cit.*, 59
155. Pfeiffer, Carl C., 1975, *op. cit.*, 165–169
156. Kamen, Betty and Si, *op. cit.*, 136

# REFERENCES

157. Jennings, I.W., *op. cit.*, 133
158. Dhopeshwarkar, Govind A., *Nutrition and Brain Development*, New York, Plenum Press, 1983, 99
159. Stempak, J.G., 'Etiology of antenatal hydrocephalus induced by folic acid deficiency in the albino rat', *Anat Rec*, 1965, 151, 287
160. Arawaka, T. et al., 'Dilation of cerebral ventricles of rat offspring induced by 6 mercapto purine administration to dams', *Tohoku J Epx Med*, 1967, 91, 143
161. Smithells, R.W. et al., 'Possible prevention of neural tube defects by preconceptual vitamin supplementation', *Lancet*, 1980, i, 339–340
162. Smithells, R.W. et al., 'Further experience of vitamin supplementation for the prevention of neural tube defect recurrences', *Lancet*, 1983, i, 1027–1031
163. Tolarova, M., 'Periconceptional supplementation with vitamins and folic acid to prevent recurrence of cleft lip', *Lancet*, ii, 217
164. Seller, Mary J., 'Prevention of neural tube defects', *The Practitioner*, 1986, 230, 719–723
165. Laurence, K.M. et al., 'Double-Blind randomised controlled trial of folate treatment before conception to prevent recurrence of neural-tube defects', *British Medical Journal*, 1981, 282, 1509–1511
166. Griffin, J.P., 'Vitamins and Neural Tube Defects', *British Medical Journal*, 1988, 296, 430
167. Nutrition Search Inc., *op. cit.*, 95
168. *Ibid*, 43
169. Marks, John, *op. cit.*, 141–143
170. Pfeiffer, Carl C., *op. cit.*, 125–138
171. Davis, Adelle, *Let's Eat Right to Keep Fit*, Unwin Paperbacks, 1971, 103–108
172. Davis, Adelle, *Let's Have Healthy Children*, Unwin Paperbacks, 1974, 26
173. Nutrition Search Inc., *op. cit.*, 96
174. Davis, Adelle, *op. cit.*, 163–169
175. Nutrition Search Inc., *op. cit.*, 63
176. Passwater, Richard A., Cranton, Elmer M., *Trace Elements, Hair Analysis and Nutrition*, New Canaan, Connecticut, Keats 1983, 31–32
177. Davis, Adelle, *op. cit.*, 143–144 and 210
178. *Ibid*, 166
179. Passwater, Richard A., *op. cit.*, 34
180. Nutrition Search Inc., *op. cit.*, 64
181. Pitkin, Roy M., 'Calcium Metabolism in Pregnancy: A Review', *Am J Obstet Gynecol*, 1975, 121, 732
182. *Ibid*, 731
183. Nutrition Search Inc., *op. cit.*, 64
184. Davis, Adelle, *op. cit.*, 163–169
185. Nutrition Search Inc., *op. cit.*, 97
186. Passwater, Richard A., *op. cit.*, 179–185
187. Underwood, Eric J., *Trace Elements in Human and Animal Nutrition*, New York, Academic Press, 1977, 152
188. *Ibid*, 151
189. Nutrition Search Inc., *op. cit.*, 67
190. Underwood, Eric J., *op. cit.*, 151
191. Nutrition Search Inc., *op. cit.*, 67
192. Underwood, Eric J., *op. cit.*, 52
193. *Ibid*, 151
194. Nutrition Search Inc., *op. cit.*, 97
195. *Ibid*, 68
196. Passwater, Richard A., *op. cit.*, 147
197. Nutrition Search Inc., *op. cit.*, 68
198. Underwood, Eric J., *op. cit.*, 83
199. *Ibid*, 75–87
200. Nutrition Search Inc., *op. cit.*, 97
201. Passwater, Richard A., *op. cit.*, 171
202. Nutrition Search Inc., *op. cit.*, 70
203. Davis, Adelle, *op. cit.*, 185
204. Pharoach, P.O.D. et al., 'Neurological damage to the fetus resulting from severe iodine deficiency during pregnancy', *Lancet*, 1971, 1, 308–310
205. Nutrition Search Inc., *op. cit.*, 70
206. Underwood, Eric J., *op. cit.*, 293–296
207. Nutrition Search Inc., *op. cit.*, 71
208. Pitkin, Roy M. et al., 'Maternal Nutrition, A Selective Review of Clinical Topics', *Obstet Gynecol*, 1972, 40, 775
209. Gibbs, C.E., Seitchik, Joseph, 'Nutrition in Pregnancy'. In: *Modern Nutrition on Health and Disease*, eds. Goodhart, Robert S. Shils, Maurice. Philadelphia, Lea and Febiger 1980, 746
210. Lesser, Michael, *op. cit.*, 132
211. Passwater, Richard A., *op. cit.*, 106
212. Nutrition Search Inc., *op. cit.*, 71
213. Davis, Adelle, *op. cit.*, 177–178
214. Watson, W.S. et al., 'Oral Absorption of Lead and Iron', *Lancet*, 1980, ii, 237
215. Oberleas, Donald, Caldwell, Donald and Prasad, Amanda, 'Trace Elements and Behaviour', *Int. review of Neurobiology*, Supp. 1972, 85.
216. Pfeiffer, Carl C., *Zinc and Other Micronutrients*, New Canaan, Connecticut, Keats 1978, 102
217. *Ibid*, 103
218. Davis, Adelle, *op. cit.*, 170
219. Pfeiffer, Carl C., 1978, *op. cit.*, 104
220. Hurley, Lucille S. et al., 'Teratogenic Effects of Magnesium Deficiency', *J Nut*, 1976, 106, 1254–1260
221. Spatling, L. and G., 'Magnesium Supplementation in pregnancy: a double-blind study'. *Br J Obstet Gynaecol*, 1988, 95, 111–116
222. Wynn, Arthur, Wynn, Margaret, *Magnesium in Pregnancy*. In press 1988
223. Nutrition Search Inc., *op. cit.*, 98
224. Williams, Roger J., 1973, *op. cit.*, 61
225. Pfeiffer, Carl C., 1978, *op. cit.*, 66
226. *Ibid*, 66
227. Underwood, Eric J., *op. cit.*, 180
228. *Ibid*, 180
229. Pfeiffer, Carl C., 1978, *op. cit.*, 72
230. Underwood, Eric J., *op. cit.*, 177
231. Oberleas & Caldwell, 1972, 88–90
232. Nutrition Search Inc., *op. cit.*, 98
233. Spears, Jerry W., 'Effect of Dietary Nickel on Growth, Urease Activity, Blood Parameters and Tissue Mineral Concentrations in the Neonatal Pig', *J Nut*, 1984, 114, 845–853
234. Underwood, Eric J., *op. cit.*, 162
235. Pfeiffer, Carl C., 1975, *op. cit.*, 301
236. Neilson, Forrest H., 'Fluoride, Vanadium, Nickel, Arsenic and Silicon in Total Parental Nutrition', *Bulletin of the New York Academy of Medicine*, 1984, 60(2), 177–195
237. Anke, M. et al., 'Nutritional Requirements of Nickel' (Offprint available through Foresight)
238. Pfeiffer, Carl C., 1978, *op. cit.*, 148–149
239. Neilson, Forrest H., 1984, *op. cit.*, 183
240. Neilson, Forrest H., 'Nickel'. In *Biochemistry of the Essential Ultratrace Elements*, ed Frieden, Earl. Plenum Publishing Corporation 1984, 299
241. Nutrition Search Inc., *op. cit.*, 77
242. Pfeiffer, Carl C., 1978, *op. cit.*, 150
243. *Ibid*, 99–101
244. Nutrition Search Inc., *op. cit.*, 77
245. Davis, Adelle, *op. cit.*, 168
246. Nutrition Search Inc., *op. cit.*, 98
247. Passwater, Richard A., *op. cit.*, 80
248. Nutrition Search Inc., *op. cit.*, 78
249. Hurley, Lucille S., *op. cit.*, 180
250. Passwater, Richard A., *op. cit.*, 82
251. Nutrition Search Inc., *op. cit.*, 79
252. *Ibid*, 98
253. Pfeiffer, Carl C., 1978, *op. cit.*, 84–89
254. Underwood, Eric J., *op. cit.*, 308
255. Pfeiffer, Carl C., 1978, *op. cit.*, 86
256. Nutrition Search Inc., *op. cit.*, 98

257. Underwood, Eric J., *op. cit.*, 401–403
258. Passwater, Richard A. *op. cit.*, 217
259. Underwood, Eric J., *op. cit.*, 391
260. Naylor, G.J. et al., 'Elevated Vanadium Content of Hair and Mania', *Biological Psychiatry*, 1984, 19(5), 759–763
261. Underwood, Eric J., *op. cit.*, 390
262. Neilson, Forrest H., *op. cit.*, 236
263. Sandstead, Harry H., 'Zinc: Essentiality for Brain Development and Function', *Nutrition Today*, 1984, November/December, 26–30
264. Pfeiffer, Carl C., 1978, *op. cit.*, 42–43
265. Crosby, Warren M. et al., 'Fetal Malnutrition: An Appraisal of Correlated Factors', *Am J Obstet Gynecol*, 1977, 128, 26
266. Sandstead, Harold H., *op. cit.*
267. Crawford, I.L., Connor, J.D., 'Zinc and Hippocampal Function', *J Orthomolecular Psych*, 1975, 4(1), 39–52
268. Caldwell, Donald F., Oberleas, Donald, 'Effects of Protein and Zinc Nutrition on Behavior in the Rat', *Perinatal Factors Affecting Human Development*, 1969, 185, 2–8
269. Pfeiffer, Carl C., 1978, *op. cit.*, 42
270. *Ibid*, 6
271. Bryce-Smith, Derek, Hodgkinson, Liz., *The Zinc Solution*, London, Century Arrow 1986, 28–29
272. Hurley, Lucille S., 'Zinc Deficiency in the Developing Rat', *Am J Clin Nut*, 1969, 22, 1332–1339
273. Underwood, Eric J., *op. cit.*, 291–220
274. Caldwell, Donald F., Oberleas, Donald, *op. cit.*
275. Bryce-Smith, Derek, *op. cit.*, 119
276. Jameson, Sten, 'Zinc Status and Human Reproduction'. In: *Zinc in Human Medicine. Proceedings of a Symposium on the Role of Zinc in Health and Disease*, 27 June 1984, Isleworth, TIL Publications Ltd. 61–80
277. Ward, N.I. et al., 'Placental Element Levels in Relation to Fetal Development for Obstetrically "Normal" Births: A Study of 37 Elements. Evidence for Effects of Cadmium, Lead, and Zinc on Fetal Growth, and Smoking as a Source of Cadmium', *Int J Biosocial Res*, 1987, 9(1), 63–81
278. Lazebnik, N. et al., 'Zinc Status, Pregnancy Complications, and Labor Abnormalities', *Am J Obstet Gynecol*, 1988, 158, 161–166
279. Jameson, Sten, *op. cit.*
280. Grant, Ellen, *The Bitter Pill*, London, Corgi, 1985, 216
281. Bryce-Smith, Derek, *op. cit.*, 119
282. Hambidge, K. Michael, et al., 'Low Levels of Zinc in Hair, Anorexia, Poor Growth, and Hypogeusia in Children', *Pediatric Research*, 1972, 6, 868–874
283. Nutrition Search Inc., *op. cit.*, 99

Chapter 6

1. Flynn, Anna, 'Natural Family Planning'. In: *Handbook of Family Planning*, London, Nancy ed. London, Churchill Livingstone, 1985, 189
2. Burger, H.G., 'The Ovulation Method', Proceedings Inter Seminar in Natural Family Planning, October 1979, Dublin, 79–90
3. Davidson, John. Davidson, Farida. *Natural Fertility Awareness*, Saffron Walden, C.W. Daniel Co Ltd., 1986
4. Wright, et al., 'Neoplasia and dysplasia of cervix uteri and contraception: a possible protective effect of the diaphragm', *Br J Cancer*, 1978, 38, 273–279
5. McEwan, John, 'Contraceptive Sponges', *Maternal and Child Health*, 1986, October, 338–341

Chapter 7

1. Lodge, Rees E., 'Trace Elements in Pregnancy', *Trace Elements in Health*, Ed J. Rose, London, Butterworths, 1983, 262
2. Ward, N.I. et al., 'Placental Element Levels in Relation to Fetal Development for Obstetrically "Normal" Births: A Study of 37 Elements. Evidence for Effects of Cadmium, Lead, and Zinc On Fetal Growth, and Smoking as a Source of Cadmium', *Int Journal of Biosocial Research*, 1987, 9(1), 63
3. Ward, N.I., Brooks, R.R., 'Lead Levels in Sheep Organs Resulting From Automotive Exhausts', *Envirn Pollut*, 1978, 17, 7–12
4. Colgan, Michael, *Your Personal Vitamin Profile*, London, Blond and Briggs, 1982, 65
5. Doctor, 24 March 1983, 76
6. Davies, Stephen, 'Lead', *Beyond Nutrition*, Summer 1981, 12–13
7. Pfeiffer, Carl C., *Zinc and Other Micronutrients*, New Canaan, Keats, 1978, 164
8. Clausen, J. and Rastogi, S.C., 'Heavy metal pollution among autoworkers. 1. Lead', *Br J Industrial Med*, 1977, 34, 208–215
9. El-Dakhakny, Abdel-Ariz, El-sadik, Yassim M., 'Lead in Hair among Exposed Workers', *Am Industrial Hygiene Assoc Journal*, 1972, 33
10. Needleman, Herbert L. et al., *JAMA*, 1984, 251(22), 2956–9
11. Elkington, John, *The Poisoned Womb*, Harmondsworth, Middlesex, Viking, 1985, 68.
12. Davies, Stephen, *op. cit.*
13. Kostial, K., Kello, Dinko, 'Bioavailability of Lead in Rats Fed "Human" Diets', *Bull Envirnm Contam Toxicol*, 1979, 21, 312–314
14. Bryce-Smith, D., Environmental Trace Elements and their Role in Disorders of Personality, Intellect, Behaviour, and Learning Ability in Children. Proceedings of the Second New Zealand Seminar on Trace Elements and Health. University of Auckland, 22–26 January 1979
15. Davies, S., *op. cit.*
16. Blumer, W., Reich, Th., 'Leaded Gasoline – A Cause of Cancer', *Environment International*, 1980, 3, 465–471
17. Davies, S., *op. cit.*
18. Schwartz, Joel et al., 'Relationship Between Childhood Blood Lead Levels and Stature', *Pediatrics*, 1986, 77(3), 281–288
19. Needleman, H.L., *op. cit.*
20. Lancranjan, I., 'Reproductive Ability of Workmen Occupationally Exposed to Lead', *Arch Environ Health*, 1975, 30, 396–401
21. Elkington, John, *op. cit.*, 113–114
22. See Reference 2 above for evidence of its accumulation
23. Wibberley, D.G. et al., 'Lead Levels in Human Placentae from Normal and Malformed Births', *J Med Genetics*, 1977, 14(5), 339–345
24. Bryce-Smith, D. et al., 'Lead and Cadmium Levels in Stillbirths', *Lancet*, 1977, i, 1159
25. Needleman, H.L., *op. cit.*
26. Singh, Nalini et al., 'Neonatal lead intoxication in a prenatally exposed infant', *J Pediatrics*, 1978, 93(6), 1019–1021
27. Bellinger, David et al., 'Low-Level Lead Exposure and Infant Development in the First Year', *Neurobehavioural Toxicol and Teratol*, 1986, 8, 151–161
28. Bellinger, David et al., 'Longitudinal Analyses of Prenatal and Postnatal Lead Exposure and Early Cognitive Development', *New Engl J Med*, 1987, 17, 1037–1043
29. Reported by Bryce-Smith, D., *op. cit.*, 14
30. Bushnell, Philip J., Bowman, Robert E., 'Reversal Learning Deficits in Young Monkeys Exposed to Lead', *Pharmacology Biochemistry and Behaviour*, 1977, 10, 733–747
31. Needleman, Herbert L. et al., 'Deficits in Psychologic and Classroom Performance of Children with Elevated Dentine Lead Levels', *New Engl J Med*, 1979, 300, 689–696

REFERENCES

32. Thatcher, R. et al., 'Effects of Low Levels of Cadmium and Lead on Cognitive Functioning in Children', *Arch Environ Health*, 1982, 37(3), 159–166
33. Garnys, V. et al., *Lead Burden of Sydney Schoolchildren*, University of New South Wales, 1979
34. Yale, W. et al., 'Teachers' Ratings of Children's Behaviour in Relation to Blood Lead Levels', *Br J of Dev Psychology*, 1985, 2, 295–306
35. Pihl, R.O., Parkes, M., 'Hair Element Content in Learning Disabled Children', *Science*, 1977, 198, 4313
36. Moore, Lewis S., Fleischman, Alan, 'Subclinical Lead Toxicity', *Orthomolecular Psychiatry*, 1975, 4(1), 61–70
37. Gittelman, Rachel, Eskenazi, Brenda, 'Lead and Hyperactivity Revisited', *Arch Gen Psychiatry*, 1983, 40, 827–833
38. Lin-Fu, J.S., 'Vulnerability of children to lead exposure and toxicity', *New Engl J Med*, 1973, 289, 1229–1233
39. David, Oliver J. et al., 'Lead and Hyperactivity. Behavioral Response to Chelation: A Pilot Study', *Am J Psychiatry*, 1976, 133(10), 1155–1158
40. Hansen, J.C. et al., 'Children with minimal brain dysfunction', *Danish Medical Bulletin*, 1980, 27(6), 259–262
41. Colgan, Michael, *op. cit.*, 63
42. Pfeiffer, Carl C., *op. cit.*, 174
43. McKie, Robin, 'Cadmium in the diet poses health danger', *Sunday Times*, 25 September 1983
44. Pfeiffer, Carl C., *op. cit.*, 174
45. Pfeiffer, Carl C., *op. cit.*, 174
46. Lappe, Mark, 'Trace Elements and the unborn: review and preliminary Implications for Policy'. In *Trace Elements in Health*. See ref 1, 237
47. Lodge Rees, Elizabeth, *op. cit.*, 263
48. Schroeder, H., Mitchener, M., 'Toxic Effects of Trace Elements on the Reproduction of mice and rats', *Arch Environ Health*, 1971, 23, 102
49. Lodge Rees, Elizabeth, *op. cit.*, 263
50. Bryce-Smith, D., Environmental Influences on Prenatal Development, Thessaloniki Conference, September 1981
51. Lodge Rees, Elizabeth, *op. cit.*, 264
52. Lodge Rees, Elizabeth, *op. cit.*, 264
53. Samarawickrama, Gervin, 'Cadmium in animal and human health'. In: *Trace Elements and Health*. See ref 1, 37
54. *Ibid*, 38
55. Kupsinel, Roy, 'Mercury Amalgam Toxicity. A Major Common Denominator of Degenerative Disease', *J Orthomolecular Psychiatry*, 13(4), 240–257
56. Elkington, John, *op. cit.*, 113
57. Elkington, John, *op. cit.*, 113
58. Kupsinel, *op. cit.*
59. Elkington, John, *op. cit.*, 71–72
60. Norwood, Christopher, *At Highest Risk*, New York, McGraw-Hill, 1980, 10–11
61. Colgan, Michael, *op. cit.*, 64
62. Pfeiffer, Carl C., *op. cit.*, 170
63. Ziff, *The Toxic Time-Bomb*, Wellingborough, Thorsons, 1985
64. Kupsinel, *op. cit.*
65. Kupsinel, *op. cit.*
66. Colgan, Michael, *op. cit.*, 65
67. *Nutrition Almanac*, New York, McGraw-Hill, 1975, 62
68. Freundlich, Michael et al., 'Infant Formula as a Cause of Aluminium Toxicity in Neonatal Uraemia', *Lancet*, 1985, ii, 527–529
69. Lodge Rees, Elizabeth, 'Aluminium Toxicity as Indicated by Hair Analysis', *J Orthomolecular Psychiatry*, 1979, 8(1), 37–43
70. Lodge Rees, Elizabeth, 1979, *op. cit.*
71. Pfeiffer, Carl C., *op. cit.*, 153–156
72. Millstone, Eric, John Abraham, *Additives. A Guide for Everyone*, London, Penguin, 1988
73. Elkington, John, *op. cit.*, 113
74. Norwood, Christopher, *op. cit.*, 102
75. Pfeiffer, Carl C., *op. cit.*, 197
76. Pfeiffer, Carl C., *op. cit.*, 198
77. Elkington, John, *op. cit.*, 113
78. Elkington, John, *op. cit.*, 117
79. Mortensen, Mary Lund et al., 'Teratology and the Epidemiology of Birth Defects'. In: Gabbe, Steven G. et al., eds. *Obstetrics. Normal and Problem Pregnancies*, New York, Churchill Livingstone, 1986, 183–210
80. Thatcher, R.W. et al., *op. cit.*
81. *Ibid*
82. Bryce-Smith, D. See ref 24
83. Bryce-Smith, D. See ref 51
84. Ward, N.I. See ref 2
85. Lester, Michael L. et al., 'Protective Effects of Zinc and Calcium Against Heavy Metal Impairment of Children's Cognitive Function', *Nutrition and Behaviour*, 1986, 2, 145–161
86. Sohler, Arthur et al., 'Blood Lead Levels in Psychiatric Outpatients Reduced by Zinc and Vitamin C', *J Orthomolecular Psychiatry*, 1977, 6(3), 272–276
87. Spivey Fox, M.R., 1975, *New York Acad Sci*, 1975, 258, 144
88. *Beyond Nutrition, op. cit.*
89. Colgan, Michael, *op. cit.*, 66
90. Kime, Zane R., *Sunlight*, Penryn, CA, World Health Publications, 1980

Chapter 8

1. Briggs, Gerald et al., *Drugs in Pregnancy and Lactation. A Reference Guide to Fetal and Neonatal Risk*, Baltimore, Williams and Wilkins, 1986. Very comprehensive
2. Broadie, Martin J., 'Drugs and Breastfeeding', *Practitioner*, 1986, 230, 483–485
3. Schelling, J.L., 'Which Drugs should not be Prescribed during Pregnancy', *Ther Umsch Rev Ther*, 1987, 441, 48–53
4. Joffe, Justin M., 'Influence of Drug Exposure of the Father on Perinatal Outcome', *Clinics in Perinatology. Symposium of Pharmacology*, 1979, 6(1), 21–36
5. Committee on Drugs, 'The Transfer of Drugs and Other Chemicals into Human Breast Milk', *Pediatrics*, 1983, 72(3), 373–383
6. Brodie, Martin J., *op. cit.*
7. Elkington, John, *The Poisoned Womb*, London, Viking, 1985, 168
8. Mann, Peggy, *Marijuana Alert*, New York, McGraw-Hill, 1985
9. Salsburg, David. In: Elkington, John, *The Poisoned Womb*, Harmondsworth, Viking, 1985, 168
10. Beaulac-Baillargeon, Louise, Desrosiers, Carole, 'Caffeine – cigarette interaction on fetal growth', *Am J Obstet Gynecol*, 1987, 157, 1236–1240
11. Mann, Peggy, *op. cit.*
12. *Ibid.*
13. Beaulac-Baillargeon, Louise, *op. cit.*
14. Buist, Robert, 'Drug-Nutrient Interactions', *International Journal of Clinical Nutrition*
15. Robertson, W.F., 'Thalidomide (Distaval) and Vitamin B Deficiency', *British Medical Journal*, 1962, 1, 792
16. Labadarios, D., 'Studies on the Effects of Drugs on Nutritional Status', 1975, Phd Thesis, University of Surrey
17. Blair, J.H. et al., 'MAO inhibitors and sperm production', *JAMA*, 1962, 181, 192–193
18. Davis, J. et al., 'Effects of phenelzine on semen in infertility: a preliminary report', *Fert Ster*, 1966, 17, 221–225
19. Collins, E., Turner, G., 'Maternal effects of regular salicylate ingestion in pregnancy', *Lancet*, 1975, 2, 335–337

20. Turner, G., Collins, E., 'Fetal effects of regular salicylate intoxification in a newborn. a case report', *Clin Pediatr* (Phila), 1976, 15, 912–913
21. Stone, D. et al., 'Aspirin and congenital malformations', *Lancet*, 1976, 1, 1373–1375
22. Shapiro, S. et al., 'Perinatal Mortality and Birthweight in Relation to Aspirin Taken During Pregnancy', *Lancet*, 1976, ii, 1375–376
23. Pyktowitz Streissgath, Ann et al., 'Aspirin and Acetaminophen Use by Pregnant Women and Subsequent Child IQ and Attention Decrements', *Teratology*, 1987, 35, 211–219
24. Fletcher, David, 'Pregnant Women being Sought for Trials with Aspirin', *Daily Telegraph*, 29 August 1988
25. Weber, L.W.D., 'Benzodiazepines in pregnancy – academical debate or teratogenic risk?', *Biological Research in Pregnancy*, 1985, 64, 151–167
26. Rodriguez, Alonso F. et al., 'Relationship between benzodiazepine ingestion during pregnancy and oral clefts in the newborn: a case-control study', *Med Clin*, 1986, 87/18, 741–743
27. Brazelton, T. Berry, 'Effect of Prenatal Drugs on the Behaviour of the Neonate', *Am J Psychiat*, 1970, 126, 1296–1303
28. Soyka, L.F., Joffe, J.M., 'Male mediated drug effects on offspring', *Prog Clin Biol Res*, 1980, 36, 49–66
29. Editorial: 'The Drugged Sperm', *British Medical Journal*, 1964, 1, 1063–1064
30. Davis, J. et al., op. cit.
31. Blair, J.H. et al, op. cit.
32. US Public Health Service, 'The Health Consequences of Smoking for Women'. A Report of the US Surgeon-General, Office on Smoking and Health, US Dept of Health and Human Services, Rockville Md, 1980
33. Simpson, W.J., 'A preliminary report on cigarette smoking and the incidence of prematurity', *Am J Obstet Gynecol*, 1957, 73, 800–815
34. Richmond, 1979
35. Crosby, W.M. et al., 'Fetal malnutrition: an appraisal of correlated factors', *Am J Obstet Gynecol*, 1977, 128, 22
36. Naeye, *JAMA*, 1979, 241
37. Grant, Ellen, 'The Effect of Smoking on Pregnancy and Children'. In: *Guidelines for Future Parents*, Witley, Surrey, 1986, 85–86
38. Abel, Ernest L., *Marihuana, Tobacco, Alcohol and Reproduction*, Boca Raton, F1, CRC Press, 1983, 31–33
39. Goujard, J., Kaminiski, C. et al., 'Maternal Smoking, Alcohol Consumption and Abruptio Placentae', *Am J Obstet Gynecol*, 1978, 130, 738
40. Himmelberger, D.U. et al., 'Cigarette smoking during pregnancy and the occurrence of spontaneous abortion and congenital abnormality', *Am J Epidemiology*, 1978, 108, 470–479
41. Fedrick, J., Anderson, A., 'Factors associated with spontaneous pre-term birth', *Br J Obstet Gynaecol*, 1976, 83, 342
42. Miller, Herbert C. et al., *Am J Obstet Gynecol*, 1976, 125, 55–60
43. Chow, Wong-Ho, 'Maternal cigarette smoking and tubal pregnancy', *Obstet Gynecol*, 1988, 71, 167–174
44. Abel, Ernest L., op. cit., 85. This gives a good overview of some of the studies in this area
45. Grant, Ellen, op. cit.
46. Mau, G., Netter, P., *Deutsche Medizinische Wochenschrift*, 1974, 99, 1113–1118
47. Grant, Ellen, op. cit.
48. *Ibid*
49. Nieburg, P. et al., 'The Fetal Tobacco Syndrome', *JAMA*, 1985, 253, 2998–2999
50. Stirling, H.F. et al., 'Passive smoking in utero: its effects on neonatal appearance', *British Medical Journal*, 1987, 295, 627–628
51. Allbut, T.C., Rolleston, H.D., A System of Medicine, 1906. Reported in: Gambling, M.D., Poisonous Brews? Letter to *Daily Telegraph*, 6 October 1987
52. Wetherall, Charles F., *Kicking the Coffee Habit*, Minneapolis, MN, 1981, 121
53. Mohsen Moussa, Mohammed, 'Caffeine and sperm motility', *Fert Ster*, 1983, 39, 845–848
54. Furuhashi, Nobuaki et al., 'Effects of Caffeine Ingestion During Pregnancy', *Gynecologic and Obstetric Investigation*, 1985, 19, 187–191
55. Wichit, Srisuphan, Bracken, Michael B., 'Caffeine consumption during pregnancy and association with late spontaneous abortion', *Am J Obstet Gynecol*, 154, 14–20
56. Saifer, Phyllis, Zellerbach, Merla, *Detox*, Ballantine Books, New York, 1984, 42–43
57. Plant, Moira. Reported in: Gill, Kerry, 'Alcohol "Safe in Pregnancy"', *The Times*, 4 November 1987
58. Kaufman, Matthew. In: Hodgkinson, Neville, 'Alcohol Threat to Babies', *Sunday Times*, 31 January 1988
59. Anderson, R.A. et al., 'Alcohol Threat to Babies', *Sunday Times*, 31 January 1988, 1
60. Kaufman, Matthew, op. cit.
61. Van Thiel, D.H., Lester, R.
62. Little, Ruth E., Sing, Scharles F., 'Father's Drinking and Infant Birth Weight: Report of an Association', *Teratology*, 1987, 36, 59–65
63. Shurygin, G.I., 'The psychogenic pathological development of personality in children and adolescents in families with fathers afflicted with alcoholism', *Zhur Nevropat i Psik*, 1978, 78, 1566–1569 (Russian)
64. Wynn, Margaret and Arthur, 'Should Men and Women Limit Alcohol Consumption when Hoping to have a Baby', The Maternity Alliance (undated)
65. Cooper, Shawn, 'The Fetal Alcohol Syndrome', *J Child Psych and Psychiat*, 1987, 28, 223–227
66. Streissguth, A.P., 'Fetal Alcohol Syndrome: Where are we in 1978?', *Women and Health*, 1979, 4, 223–237
67. Rosett, H.L. et al., 'Patterns of Alcohol Consumption and Fetal Development', *Obstet Gynecol*, 1983, 61, 539–546
68. Cooper, Shawn., op. cit.
69. Anon., *Boston Globe*, 11 February 1987
70. Mann, Peggy, op. cit., 8
71. Elam, Daniel, *Building Better Babies. Preconception Planning for Healthier Children*, Millbrae, CA, Celestial Arts, 1980
72. Issidorides, Marietta. In: Mann, Peggy, op. cit., 167–169
73. Morishama, Akira. In: Mann, Peggy, op. cit., 202–203
74. Sassenrath, E.N. et al., 'Reproduction in Rhesus Monkeys Chronically Exposed to Delta-9-THC', *Advances in the Biosciences*, 1979, 22–23, 501–522
75. Stenchever, M.A. et al., 'Chromosome Breakages in Users of Marijuana', *Am J Obstet Gynecol*, 1974, 118, 106–113
76. Mann, Peggy, op. cit.
77. Mahalik, M.P. et al., 'Teratogenic potential of cocaine hydrochloride in CF-1 mice', *J Pharm Sci*, 1980, 69, 703–706
78. Fantel, A.G., Macphail, B.J., 'The teratogenicity of cocaine', *Teratology*, 1982, 26, 17–19
79. Bongol, Nesrin et al., 'Teratogenicity of cocaine in humans', *J Pediatr*, 1987, 1, 93–96
80. Smith, Carole Grace, Gilbean, Pamela M., 'Drug Abuse Effects on Reproductive Hormones'. In: *Endocrine Toxicology*, ed Thomas, J. et al., New York, Raven Press, 1985

REFERENCES

81. Ostrea, E.M., Chavez, C.J., 'Perinatal problems (excluding neonatal withdrawal) in maternal drug addiction: a study of 830 cases', *J Pediatr*, 1979, 94, 292–295
82. Naeye, R.L. et al., 'Fetal Complications of Maternal Heroin Addiction: Abnormal Growth, Infections and Episodes of Stress', *J Pediatr*, 1973, 83, 1055–1061
83. Wilson, G.S. et al., 'The development of preschool children of heroin addicted mothers: a controlled study', *Pediatrics*, 1979, 63, 135–141
84. Keller Phelps, Janice, Morse, Alan, *The Hidden Addiction*, Boston, Little Brown and Company, 1986
85. Royal College of Psychiatrists. Drug Scenes. A Report on Drugs and Drug Dependence by the Royal College of Psychiatrists, London, Gaskell, 1985
86. Keller Phelps, Janice, *op. cit.*

Chapter 9

1. Grant, Ellen, Personal Communication, April 1988
2. Royal College of General Practitioners, *Oral Contraceptives and Health*, London, Pitman Medical Books, 1974
3. Kays, Clifford, 'The RCPG's Oral Contraceptive Study: Some Recent Observations', *Clinics in Obstetrics and Gynaecology*, 1984, 11, 3
4. Grant, Ellen, *The Bitter Pill*, London, Corgi, 1985
5. *Op. cit.*, 106
6. *Op. cit.*, 108
7. Dankenbring, William F., *Your Keys to Radiant Health*, New Canaan, Connecticut, Keats Publishing, 1974
8. Williams, Harold, *The Pill in New Perspective: Pregnant or Dead?*, New Perspective Publications, San Francisco, 1969, 69. Mentioned in ref 6 above, 76
9. Seamans, Barbara. In ref 6 above, 77
10. Airola, Paavo, *Every Woman's Health*, Phoenix, Arizona, Health Plus Publishers, 1979, 322–323
11. Grant, Ellen, *op. cit.*
12. Grant, Ellen, Personal Communication, April 1988
13. ORTHO-NOVIN* 1/50 Oral Contraceptive Tablets. Instruction sheet
14. Grant, *op. cit.*, 215–219
15. Grant, *op. cit.*, 218
16. Polan, Mary Lake, 'Ectopic Pregnancy'. In: *Reproductive Failure*, ed. Alan H. DeCherney, New York, Churchill Livingstone, 1986, 257
17. Grant, Ellen, Personal Communication, April 1988
18. Grant, *op. cit.*, 77–100
19. Grant, *op. cit.*, 121
20. Gal, I. et al., 'Hormonal pregnancy tests and congenital malformations', *Nature*, 1967, 216, 83
21. Harlap, Susan et al., 'Congenital Abnormalities in the Offspring of Women Who Used Oral and Other Contraceptives Around the Time of Conception', *Int J Fertil*, 1985, 30, 39–47
22. Royal College of General Practitioners, 'The Outcome of Pregnancy on Former Oral Contraceptive Users', *Br J Obstet Gynaecol*, 1976, 83, 608–616
23. Nora, Audrey and Nora, James J., 'A Syndrome of Multiple Congenital Anomalies Associated with Teratogenic Exposure', *Arch Evirn Health*, 1975, 30, 17–21
24. Nora, J.J., et al., 'Exogenous progestogen and estrogen implicated in birth defects', *J Am Med Ass*, 1978, 240(9), 837
25. Hellstrom, B. et al., 'Prenatal sex-hormone exposure and congenital limb reduction Anomalies', *Lancet*, 1976, 2, 372–373
26. Janerich, D.T. et al., 'Oral contraceptives and congenital limb reduction defects', *N Eng J Med*, 1974, 291 (ii), 697–700
27. McCreadie, J. et al., 'Congenital Limb Defects and the Pill', *Lancet*, 1983, 2, 623
28. Kricker, Anne et al., 'Congenital limb reduction deformities and use of oral contraceptives', *Am J Obstet Gynecol*, 1986, 155, 1072–1078
29. Levy, E.P. et al., 'Hormone treatment during pregnancy and congenital heart defects', *Lancet*, 1973, 1, 611
30. Mullvihill, J.J. et al., 'Congenital Heart Defects and Prenatal Sex Hormones', *Lancet*, 1974, 1, 1168
31. Oakley, G.P. et al., 'Hormonal pregnancy tests and congenital malformations', *Lancet*, 1973, 2, 256–257
32. Airola, *op. cit.*, 329–330

Chapter 10

1. Spyker, Joan M., 'Occupational Hazards and the Pregnant Worker', *Behavioral Toxicology Overview*, 470
2. Bertell, Rosalie. In: Toynbee, Polly, 'Behind the Lines', *Guardian*, 15 December 1986, 12
3. *Dispatches*, Channel 4 TV, 8 January 1988
4. Bertell, Rosalie, *op. cit.*
5. Ferreira, Antonio J., *Prenatal Environmental*, Springfield, Ill, Charles C. Thomas, 1969
6. Bithell, J.F., Stewart, A.M., 'Prenatal irradiation and childhood malignancy: a review of British data from the Oxford Survey', *Br J Cancer*, 1975, 31, 271–287
7. Nomura, T., 'Parental exposure to X-Rays and chemicals induces heritable tumours and anomalies in mice', *Nature*, 1982, 296, 575–577
8. Kirk, K.M., Lyon, M.F., 'Induction of congenital malformations in the offspring of male mice treated with X-Rays at pre-meiotic and post-meiotic stages', *Mutation Research*, 1984, 125, 75-85
9. McCree, Donald. In: Gold, Michael, 'Additional findings at low exposures have prompted serious second thoughts about US safeguards', *Science 80*, Premier Issue, 81
10. Hollwich, Fritz, *The Influence of Ocular Light Perception on Metabolism in Man and Animals*, New York, Springer-Verlag, 1980, Preface
11. Ott, John N., *Light, Radiation and You*, Greenwich, CN, 1985, 78–139. These two chapters give some interesting examples
12. Gabby, Samuel Lee, 'Observations on the effects of artificial light on the health and development of mice'. In: Ott, John N., *op. cit.*, 100
13. Rosenthal, Norman E. et al., 'Antidepressant Effects of Light in Seasonal Affective Disorder', *Am J Psychiatr*, 1985, 2, 163–170
14. Mayron, Lewis W. et al., 'Light, Radiation and Academic Behavior', *Academic Therapy*, 1974, X(1), 33–47
15. Kime, Zane R., *Sunlight*, Penryn, World Health Publications, 1980, 199
16. McCarthy, Paul, *Health*, February 1988, 32
17. Kime, Zane R., *op. cit.*, 92
18. *Ibid*, 92–3
19. *Ibid*, 244–245
20. *Ibid*, 162
21. *Ibid*, 200
22. Bonnell, J.A., 'Physical Hazards'. In: Dizon, W.M., Price, Susan M.G., eds. *Aspects of Occupational Health*, Faber and Faber, 1984, 167–194

23. Webb, Tony. Reported in: Stuttaford, Thomas, 'The Screen of Fear', Medical Briefing, *The Times*, 15 November 1984
24. *Ibid*
25. Anon., 'Microwaves. The Invisible Danger to Expectant Mums', *Healthy Living*, 12 March 1985
26. Anon., CIP Bulletin, St Louis, MO, 12 July 1980
27. Schauss, Alexander G., Body Chemistry and Human Behaviour. Course: Oxford, 18 November 1986
28. Stellman, Jeanne, Daum, Susan M., *Work is Dangerous to your Health*, Vintage Books, 1979, 141
29. Wright, Pearce, 'Claims that power cables cause Cancer to be investigated', *The Times*, 18 March 1988
30. Anon., 'Power Lines Cancer Link', *Today*, 18 March 1988
31. Nordstrom, S. et al., 'Reproductive hazards among workers at high-voltage systems', *Bioelectromagnetics*, 1981, 4, 91–101
32. Wertheimer, N., Leeper, E., Adverse effects on fetal development associated with sources of exposure to 60 Hz electric and magnetic fields. (Abstract) 23rd Hanford Life Sciences Symposium. Interaction of Biological Systems with Static and ELF Electric and Magnetic Fields. Richland, W.A., 1984
33. Andrews, Lori B., *New Conceptions*, New York, St Martin's Press, 1984, 23
34. Teymor, Melvin L., *Infertility*, New York, Grune and Stratton Inc, 1978
35. *Ibid*
36. Smith, David W., *Mothering Your Unborn Baby*, Philadelphia, W.B. Saunders, 1979, 67
37. Polakoff, Phillip L., *Work and Health. It's Your Life*, Washington, Press Associates Inc, 1984
38. Ferreira, Antonio J., op. cit., 59–60
39. Stuttaford, Thomas, 'Listening In', *The Times*, 21 July 1988
40. Spyker, Joan, op. cit., 471
41. Spyker, Joan, op. cit., 471
42. Kapp, Robert W. et al., 'Y-Chromosomal Nondisjunction in Dibromochloropropane-Exposed Workmen', *Mutation Research*, 1979, 64, 47–51
43. Norwood, Christopher, *At Highest Risk*, New York, McGraw-Hill, 1980, 190
44. Elkington, John, *The Poisoned Womb*, Harmondsworth, Middx, Viking, 1985, 63
45. *Ibid*, 231
46. Barlow, S.M., Sullivan, F.M., *Reproductive Hazards of Industrial Chemicals*, London, Academic Press Inc, 1982, 40
47. Mortensen, Mary Lund, et al., 'Teratology and the Epidemiology of Birth Defects'. In: Gabbe, Stephen G. et al., eds. *Obstetrics, Normal and Problem Pregnancies*, New York, Churchill Livingstone, 1986, 201
48. Norwood, Christopher, op. cit.,192
49. Elkington, John, op. cit., 72
50. *Ibid*, 117
51. Barlow, S.M., op. cit., 40–41
52. Barlow, S.M., *Ibid*, 40–41
53. Barlow, S.M., *Ibid*, 40–41
54. Stellman, Jeanne M., op. cit., 190
55. Barlow, S.M., op. cit., 41
56. Chavkin, Wendy, ed. 'Double Exposure. Women's Health Hazards – on the Job and at Home', New York, *Monthly Review Press*, 1984, 190
57. *Lancet*, 1987, 2, 1153
58. Greenpeace, *Stepping Lightly on the Earth*, undated
59. McDowall, M.E., 'OPCS Occupational Reproductive Epidemiology: The Use of Routinely Collected Statistics in England and Wales 1980–1982', *Studies on Medical and Population Subjects No 50*, London, HMSO 1985
60. Nicholson-Lord, 'Eye Damage Risk in "Sick" Offices', *The Times*, 12 March 1988
61. Fletcher, David, 'Scourge of the Sick Building Syndrome', *The Daily Telegraph*, 24 March 1988
62. Norwood, Christopher, op. cit., 47
63. *Ibid*, 39
64. *Ibid*, 40–41
65. *Ibid*, 40

Chapter 11

1. Balfour, E.B., *The Living Soil and the Haughey Experiment*, New York, Universe Books, 1976, 29
2. Bunyard, Peter, Morgan-Grenville, Fern, eds. *The Green Alternative*, London, Methuen, 1987, 83
3. Garraway, James L., 'Trace Elements in Agriculture', *Trace Elements in Health*, Rose, J., ed. London, Butterworth
4. Mansfield, Peter, Monro, Jean, *Chemical Children*, London, Century 1987, 31
5. Garraway, James L., op. cit.
6. Bryce-Smith, Derek, Hodgkinson, Liz, *The Zinc Solution*, London, Century Arrow 1986, 33–38
7. Pfeiffer, Carl C., *Mental and Elemental Health*, New Canaan, Connecticut, Keats 1975, 256
8. Vogtmann, H., 'The Quality of Agricultural Produce Originating from Different Systems of Cultivation'. Bristol, The Soil Association Ltd. Translation of a paper by Vogtmann, written in 1979
9. Socialist Countryside Group, *The Seed Scandal*, Sevenoaks Socialist Countryside Group 1987
10. *Ibid*
11. Bunyard, Peter, Morgan-Grenville, Fern, eds., op. cit., 99
12. Duffy, Frank H., Burchfield, James L., 'Long Term Effects of the Organophosphate Sarin on EEGs in Monkeys and Humans', *Neurotoxicology*, 1980, 1, 667–689
13. *Ibid*
14. *Gray's Anatomy*, 1954, 908
15. Roberts, D., 'Pharmacology and Toxicology of Organophosphorus Pesticides' (Offprint available from Foresight)
16. Duffy, Frank H., op. cit., 668
17. Duffy, Frank H. et al., 'Long-term Effects of an Organophosphate upon the Human Electroencephalogram', *Toxicology and Applied Pharmacology*, 1979, 47, 161–176
18. Roberts, D., op. cit., 198–206
19. Johnson, M.K., 'The Delayed Neuropathy Caused by Some Organophosphorus Esters: Mechanism and Challenge', *CRC Critical Reviews in Toxicology*, June 1975, 289–313
20. Andrews, A.H., 'Abnormal reactions and their frequency in cattle following the use of organophosphorus warble fly dressing', *The Veterinary Record*, 1981, 109, 171–175
21. Purdy, M., Personal Communication
22. Anon., 'Garden Weedkillers Ban', *The Daily Telegraph*, 9 March 1988
23. Young, Robin, 'Pesticide found in a third of fresh fruit', *The Times*, 16 April 1988
24. Erlichman, James, *Gluttons for Punishment*, London, Penguin 1986, 24
25. Hill, Stuart B., Soil Conditions and Food Quality. Undated paper by author, MacDonald College of McGill University
26. Ramsay Tainsh, A., Mycotoxicosis and Birth Defects. Paper dated 15 May 1984
27. Schoental, Regina, 'Mycotoxins'. In: *Guidelines for Future Parents*, Foresight, October 1986
28. Erlichman, James, op. cit., 25
29. Hill, Stuart B., op. cit.

REFERENCES

30. Powledge, Fred, *Fat of the Land*, New York, Simon and Schuster, 1984, 44
31. Colgan, Michael, *Your Personal Vitamin Profile*, London, Blond and Briggs, 1982, 35
32. Erlichman, James, *op. cit.*, 17
33. *Ibid*, 19
34. *Ibid*, 50–53
35. *Ibid*, 40
36. *Ibid*, 109
37. Schell, Orville, *Modern Meat*, New York, Random House, 1978, 176
38. 'Profits fall at Bernard Matthews', *The Times*, 24 March 1988
39. Powledge, Fred, *Ibid*, 44
40. See Cannon, Geoffrey, Walker, Caroline, *The Food Scandal*, London, Century Arrow, 1986, 121–154 for an excellent exposé of processed meat products
41. *Ibid*
42. National Advisory Committee on Nutrition Education. Proposals for Nutritional Guidelines for Health Education in Britain. Health Education Council, 1983, 23
43. Davis, Donald R., 'Wheat and Nutrition', *Nutrition Today*, 1981, 16(4)
44. Schroeder, Henry A., *The Trace Elements and Man*, Old Greenwich, Devin-Adair, 1973, 152
45. Brady, Margaret, 'Food for Prospective Parents, Bread for Health and Vitality'. In: ref 27 above, 45
46. Williams, Roger J., *Nutrition Against Disease*, New York, Bantam, 1971, 205
47. Ballentine, Rudolph, *Diet and Nutrition*, Honesdale, P.A., The Himalayan International Institute, 1978, 72
48. *Ibid*, 250
49. Jervis, Ruth and Norman, *The Foresight Wholefood Cookbook*, London, Roberts Publications, 1984, 103
50. Yudkin, J., *Pure, White and Deadly*, London, Viking, 1986
51. Lester, John, Personal Communication
52. Keller Phelps, Janice, Norse, Alan E., *The Hidden Addiction and How to Get Free*, Boston, Little Brown and Company 1986, 73
53. Ballentine, Rudolph, *op. cit.*, 56
54. Schroeder, Henry A., *op. cit.*, 152
55. Colgan, Michael, *op. cit.*, 35
56. Millstone, Erik, Abraham, John, *Additives. A Guide for Everyone*, London, Penguin, 1988, 11
57. *Ibid*, 11
58. Cannon, Geoffrey, *The Politics of Food*, London, Century, 1987. This is an excellent review of the food scene in the UK, with very comprehensive chapters on sugars, additives and other aspects.
59. Anon., *Find Out*, Foresight, 1986
60. Anon., Food Irradiation Facts, National Coalition to Stop Food Irradiation, San Francisco, CA, undated
61. Anon., *About Food Irradiation*, Bread and Circus, Boston, MA, 1987
62. Webb, Tony, Food Irradiation in Britain? London Food Commission, 1985
63. Kenton, Leslie and Susannah, *Raw Energy*, London, Century 1984, 32
64. *Ibid*, 34
65. Howell, Edward, *Food Enzymes for Health and Longevity*, Woodstock Valley, Connecticut, Omangod Press, 1980, 5
66. Kenton, Leslie, *op. cit.*, 36
67. *Ibid*, 35
68. *Ibid*, 36
69. Ballentine, Rudolph, *op. cit.*, 462

Chapter 12

1. Von Pirquet, Clement, 1906
2. Hare, Francis, *The Food Factor in Disease*, 1905
3. 'Food Allergy: How Much in the Mind', *Lancet*, 1983, 1, 1259–1261
4. Masefield, Jennifer, 'Psychiatric Illness caused or exacerbated by Food Allergies', 1988 (Unpublished paper)
5. Anon., Oregon Enacts America's First Law to Diagnose Underlying Organic Causes of Mental Illness, *Int J Biosocial Res*, 1984, 6(1), 13
6. Grant, E.C.G., Food Allergies and Migraine, *Lancet*, 1979, 1, 966–968
7. Egger, J. et al., 'Controlled Trial of Oliantigenic Treatment in the Hyperkinetic Syndrome', *Lancet*, 1985, 1, 540–545
8. *Ibid*
9. Foresight, *Guidelines for Future Parents*, 55
10. Eagle, Robert, *Eating and Allergy*, Wellingborough, Thorsons, 1986. This book gives an excellent survey of food allergy, including useful sections on diagnosis and desensitisation
11. Mansfield, Peter, Munro, Jean, *Chemical Children*, London, Century, 1987. This book gives an overview of how harmful pollutants, including chemicals, can affect children
12. Bryce-Smith, D., Simpson, R.I.D., 'Anorexia, Depression, and Zinc Deficiency', *Lancet*, 1984, ii, 1162
13. Bryce-Smith, Derek, Hodgkinson, Liz, *The Zinc Solution*, London, Century Arrow, 1986, 53–57. These pages give a brief overview of the history of anorexia and its conventional treatment
14. *Ibid*, 73
15. *Ibid*, 79
16. *Ibid*, 88
17. *Ibid*, 89
18. *Ibid*, 125–128
19. Pfeiffer, Carl C., *Zinc and other Micronutrients*, New Canaan, Keats, 1978, 197–198
20. Eagle, Robert, *op. cit.*, 115

Chapter 13

1. Rhodes, A.J., Virus Infections and Congenital Malformations. Congenital malformations: papers and discussions presented at the First International Conference on Congenital Malformations. Philadephia-Lippincott, 1961
2. Fine, P.E.M. et al., 'Infectious Diseases During Pregnancy. A follow-up study of the long-term effects of exposure to viral infections *in utero*. Studies on Medical and Population Subjects', HMSO, 1985
3. Alkalay, Arie L. et al., 'Fetal varicella syndrome', *J Paediatrics*, 1987, III 3, 320–323
4. Brunell, P.A., 'Varicella-Zoster infections in pregnancy', *JAMA*, 1967, 199, 315–354
5. Savage, Mo, et al., 'Maternal Varicella Infection as a Cause of Fetal Malformations', *Lancet*, 1973, 1, 352–354
6. Sutton, Grahame, Personal Communication, April 1988
7. Aspock, H., Toxoplasmosis. In: Prenatal and perinatal infections, EURO Reports and Studies, 93, 43–51
8. Taylor-Robinson, D., *Infertility in Infections and Pregnancy*, Ed by C.R. Coid, London, Academic Press, 1977, 141–206
9. Alder, Michael W., *ABC of Sexually Transmitted Diseases*, London, BMA, 1984, 48
10. Elek, S.D., Stern, H., 'Development of a vaccine against mental retardation caused by cytomegalovirus infection *in utero*', *Lancet*, 1974, 1, 1–5
11. Hanshaw, J.B., 'Developmental abnormalities associated with congenital cytomegalovirus infection', *Adv Teratology*, 1970, 4, 62

12. Dahle, A.J. et al., 'Progressive hearing impairment in children with congenital cytomegalovirus infection', *J Speech Hear Dis*, 1979, 44, 220
13. Blattner, Russell J., 'The Role of Viruses in Congenital Defects', *Am J Dis Child*, 1974, 128, 781–786
14. Fine, *op. cit.*
15. e.g. Grant, Ellen, Personal Communication, April 1988
16. Truss, C. Orion, *Missing Diagnosis*, MD, Inc, 1983
17. Crook, William G., *The Yeast Connection*, Professional Books, 1983
18. Davies, Stephen and Stewart, Alan, *Nutritional Medicine*, London, Pan, 1987, 360
19. Hurley, Rosalind. Reported in: Davies, S., *op. cit.*, 364
20. Schachter, Julius and Grossman, Moses, 'Chlamydia'. In: *Infectious Diseases of the Fetus and Newborn Infant*, Jack Remington and Jerome O. Klein, eds. W.B. Saunders Co, 1983
21. Ibid
22. Mardh, P.H., 'Medical Chlamydiology – A Position Paper', *Scandinavian Journal of Infectious Diseases* (Supp 32), 1981, 3–8
23. Mardh, P.A. et al., 'Endometriosis caused by Chlamydia Trachomatis', *Br J Vener Dis*, 1981, 57, 191
24. Henry-Suchat et al., 'Microbiology of Specimens obtained by laparoscopy from controls and from patients with pelvic inflammatory disease or infertility with tubal obstruction: chlamydia trachomatis and ureaplasma urealyticum', *Am J Obstet Gynecol*, 1980, 138, 1022
25. Eilard, T. et al., 'Isolation of Chlamydia in acute salpingitis', *Scandinavian Journal of Infectious Diseases* (Suppl 9), 1976, 82–84
26. Moore, D.E., et al., 'Association of chlamydia trachomatis with tubal infertility', *Fert Ster*, 1980, 34, 303–304
27. Munday, P.E., 'Chlamydial Infection'. In: *Progress in Obstetrics and Gynaecology*, 3, 1983, 231–245
28. Fromell, George T. et al., 'Chlamydial infections of mothers and their infants', *J Ped 1979*, 95(1), 28–32
29. Schachter, J. et al., 'Prospective Study of Chlamydial Infection in Neonates', *Lancet*, 1979, 2, 377–380
30. Schaefer, Catherine, et al., 'Illness in Infants Born to Women with Chlamydia Trachomatis Infection', *Am J Diseases of Children*, 1985, 139, 127–133
31. Solletico, D. et al., 'Prenatal Chlamydial Trachomatis Infection with Postnatal Respiratory Disease in a Preterm Infant', *Acta Paediatr Scan*, 1987, 76, 932
32. Cherry, Sheldon H., *Planning Ahead for Pregnancy*, London, Viking, 1987, 75
33. Brooks, Geoffrey F., 'Neisseria gonorrhoea infections in children'. In: *Gonococcal Infections*, Geoffrey F. Brooks and Elizabeth A. Donegan, eds. E. Arnold, 1985, 132
34. Israel, K.S. et al., 'Neonatal and childhood gonococcal infections', *Clin Obs Gyn*, 1975, 18, 143–151
35. Brooks, *op. cit.*, 133–134
36. Scarrel, P.M., Pratt, K.A., 'Symptomatic gonorrhea during pregnancy', *Obstet Gynaecol*, 1968, 32, 670–673
37. Health Education Council, 'Herpes. What It Is, and How to Cope', Health Education Council, 1985
38. Ibid
39. Sacks, Stephen L., *The Truth about Herpes*, Vancouver, Verdant Press, 1986, 87
40. Ibid, 82
41. Brown, Zane A. et al., 'Effects on Infants of a First Episode of Genital Herpes during pregnancy', *New Eng J Med*, 1987, 317, 1246–1251
42. Sacks, *op. cit.*, 78–80
43. Sacks, *op. cit.*, 49
44. Schofield, C.B.S., *Sexually Transmitted Diseases*, London, Churchill Livingstone, 1972
45. Ibid
46. Ibid
47. Cassell, Gail, ed. 'Ureaplasmas of humans: with emphasis on maternal and neonatal infections', *Pediatric Infectious Disease*, 1986, 5, 6, Suppl.
48. Sutton, Grahame, 'Genital Infection', *Midwife, Health Visitor and Community Nurse*, 1982, 18(2), 42–45
49. Walton, Pauline, 'New antibiotics in fight against genital disease', *Doctor*, 11 September, 1980, 39
50. Grant, Ellen, Personal Communication, April 1988
51. Friberg, J., Gnarpe, H., 'Mycoplasma and human reproductive failure', *Am J Obstet Gynecol*, 1973, 116, 23–26
52. Gibbs, Ronald S., 'Microbiology of the female genital tract', *Am J Obstet and Gynecol*, 1987, 156, 491–495
53. Simpson, Joe Leigh, 'Fetal Wastage'. In: *Obstetrics, Normal and Problem Pregnancies*, Gabbe, Steven, et al, eds. New York, Churchill Livingstone, 1986, 665
54. Sutton, Grahame, *op. cit.*
55. Sutton, Grahame, *op. cit.*
56. Jacob, Martha, et al., 'A forgotten factor in pelvic inflammatory disease: infection in the male partner', *British Medical Journal*, 1987, 294, 869
57. Grant, Ellen, *The Bitter Pill*, London, Corgi, 1975, 174
58. Westrom, L., 'Effect of acute pelvic infectious disease on fertility', *Am J Obstet Gynecol*, 1975, 121, 707–713
59. Catterall, R.D., 'Biological Effects of Sexual Freedom', *Lancet*, 1981, 1, 315–319
60. Health Education Council. Guide to a Healthy Sex Life, 1985, 22
61. Hollingworth, Barton, et al., 'Colposcopy of women with cervical HPV type 16 infection but normal cytology', *Lancet*, 1987, 2, 1148
62. Corbett, Margaret-Ann and Jerrilyn. H. Meyer, *The Adolescent and Pregnancy*, 1987, Boston, Oxford, Blackwell Scientific Publications, 1987
63. Dulfer, Susan, 'Hepatitis B and the newborn: a case for vaccination', *Maternal and Child Health*, 1987, 12, 206–212
64. Grant, *op. cit.*, 178
65. Gibbs, Ronald S. *op. cit.*
66. Hardy, P.H. et al., 'Prevalence of six sexually transmitted disease agents among pregnant inner-city adolescents and pregnancy outcome', *Lancet*, 1984, 2, 333–337
67. Schneider, A. et al., 'Colposcopy is Superior to Cytology for the Detection of Early Genital Human Papillomavirus Infection', *Obstet Gynaecol*, 1988, 71, 236–241
68. Sutton, Grahame, Personal Communication
69. Walker, Isobel, 'The symptomless sex disease', *Independent*, 24 November 1987
70. Grant, Ellen, Personal Communication, April 1988

Chapter 14

1. McNay, M.B., 'Diagnostic ultrasonography', *Clin Obstet and Gynaec*, 1987, 1, 1
2. Pearce, J. Malcolm, 'Making waves: current controversies in obstetric ultrasound', *Midwifery*, 1987, 3, 25–38
3. Dixon, H.G., *Obstetrics and Gynaecology*, London, Wright, 1980
4. Harris, R., Read, A.P., 'New uncertainties in Pre-natal Screening for Neural Tube Defect, *British Medical Journal*, 19, 282, 1416–1418

REFERENCES

5. Sutton, Grahame, Personal Communication, April 1988
6. American College of Radiology, 'Diagnostic Ultrasound in Obstetrics and Gynecology', *Tech Bull*, No 63, October 1981
7. National Center for Devices and Radiological Health of the Food and Drug Administration of USA, FDA Pub No 82–8190, 1982
8. Crum, L.A., Fowlkes, J.B., 'Acoustic cavitation generated by microsecond pulses of ultrasound', *Nature*, 1986, 319, 2 January 1986
9. Haire, D., Fetal Effects of Ultrasound: A Growing Controversy. International Society of Psychosomatic Obstetrics and Gynaecology, 7th International Congress, 14–15 September, 1983
10. Finkel, M.J., National Foundation/March of Dimes Symposium on Drug and Chemical Risks to the Fetus and Newborn Infant, New York City, 21 May 1979
11. Consumers Association, Drug and Therapeutics Bulletin, July 1985, 23, 15
12. Loeffler, F.E.. 'Chorionic villus biopsy'. In *Progress in Obstetrics and Gynaecology*, Volume 5, John Studd ed. Edinburgh, Churchill Livingstone, 1985, 22–35
13. Liu, D.T.Y. et al., 'A prospective study of spontaneous miscarriage in ultrasonically normal pregnancies and relevance to chorion villus sampling', *Prenatal Diagnosis*, 1987, 7, 223–227
14. Lilford, Richard J., 'Chorion Villus Biopsy', *Maternal and Child Health*, 1985, 198–202
15. Brook, D.J.H., *Early Diagnosis of Fetal Defects*, Churchill Livingstone, 1982, 118
16. Ager, R.P., Oliver, R.W.A., The Risks of Midtrimester Amniocentesis. Biological Materials Analysis Research Unit, University of Salford. 1986, 158
17. *Ibid*, 196
18. Turnbull, A.C., 'Amniocentesis'. In: *Antenatal and Neonatal Screening*, Wald, N.J., ed. 1984, Oxford, Oxford University Press, 1984, 445–465
19. Ager and Oliver, *op. cit.*, 159
20. Medical Research Council Working Party on Amniocentesis, 'An Assessment of the Hazards of Amniocentesis', *Br J Obstet Gynaec*, 1978, 85, suppl 2, 1–41
21. Ritchie, J.W.K., Thompson, W., 'A Critical Review of Amniocentesis in Clinical Practice'. In: Bonner, John, ed. *Recent Advances in Obstetrics and Gynaecology*, 14, Edinburgh, Churchill Livingstone, 1982, 47–70

Index

abortions, 36, 154, 157–8
addiction, drug, 100–1
additives, food, 92, 131–2
adrenal stress, 52
aflotoxin, 133
age, and infertility, 39
Ager, 158
agriculture: food production, 122–8
   hazards, 120
   organic farming, 122, 123, 124
   soil, 122
AIDS, 152
air pollution, 92
Airola, Dr Paavo, 105
airports, hazards, 120
alcohol, 22, 93, 94 98–9, 102
algin, 91
allergies, 12–13, 22, 28, 135–40
   hair mineral analysis, 52
   and the pill, 108
alpha fetoprotein, 155
aluminium: food packaging, 133
   hair mineral analysis, 51
   kitchenware, 92
   poisoning, 82, 88
Alzheimer's disease, 82, 88
American College of Radiology, 156
American Foundation for Maternal and Child Health, 156
American Society of Anesthesiologists, 119
American Society of Dental Surgeons, 87
amino acids, 58, 134
amniocentesis, 32, 157–8
animal production, 127–8
anorexia nervosa 140–2
antibiotics, 127–8, 147–8
antibodies, 15, 135
anti-convulsants, 95
anti-depressants, 95
antimony, 90
arachidonic acid, 62
arsenic, 51, 89, 90
artifical insemination (AID), 40
aspermine, 58
aspirin, 93, 95
Association of Public Analysts, 126
asthma, 135

B-complex vitamins, 62–5, 91
bacteria: food irradiation, 132–3
   sexually transmitted diseases, 147
Balfour, Lady Eve, 122
Barrett, Dr, 50–1
barrier methods, contraception, 79–80
basal temperature, 48
benzene, 111, 118
benzodiazepines, 96
Berry, Dr, 85
Bertell, Dr Rosalie, 112
beta-blockers, 96
biochemical individuality, 56
biotin, 65–6
Bircher-Benner, Max, 133
birth weight, low, 90
blood pressure tests, 48, 154
blood tests, 48, 154
Body, Sir Richard, 117
botulism, 133
brain, lead damage, 85
breast cancer, 115
breastfeeding, 117, 143
British Medical Association (BMA), 54–5, 133
British Medical Journal, 105
bromoxynil, 126
Bryce-Smith, Professor, 82, 89–90, 140–1
bulimia nervosa, 140–2

cadmium: from smoking, 96
   hair mineral analysis, 51
   and infertility, 24, 25
   poisoning, 82, 86, 89–91
   in white flour, 130
caffeine, 94, 97–8, 102
calcium: deficiency, 52
   functions and sources, 69
   hair mineral analysis, 52
   protective effect against toxic metals, 90–1
Caldwell, Donald, 57
cancer: breast, 115
   cervical, 108, 151–2
   skin, 114
   testicular, 15

INDEX

candida albicans, 23, 52
candidiasis, 147–8, 153
cannabis, 99–100
caps, contraceptive, 79–80
carbohydrates, 58
carbon monoxide, 97, 99
carotene, 60
Carson, Rachel, 125
case histories, 20–32
Catterall, 151
cavitation, ultrasound scanning, 156
Center for Disease Control, 84
Central Electricity Generating Board, 115
cereals, 126–7, 129–30
cervical caps, 79
cervix, 37
   cancer, 108, 151–2
   natural family planning, 77, 78
chemicals, occupational hazards, 111, 116–18
chickenpox, 145–6
children: hyperactivity, 85
   learning difficulties, 43, 85
chlamydia, 14–15, 39, 148–9, 153
chloramphenicol, 127
chlorinated pesticides, 117
chloroprene, 118
cholesterol, 114
choline, 65
cholinesterase, 125
chorion villus biopsy, 156–7
chromium: deficiency, 52
   detoxification with, 91
   functions and sources, 69
   hair mineral analysis, 52
chromosomal aberrations, 47
cigarette smoking, 83, 93, 94, 96–7, 102
cleaners, domestic, 118
cleft palate, 29
clingfilm, 133
Clomid, 15, 24
club feet, 30–1
cobalt: deficiency, 52
   functions and sources, 69–70
   hair mineral analysis, 52
coca-cola, 93
cocaine, 100
codeine, 100
coeliac condition, 140
coffee, 93, 97
coils (intra-uterine devices), 109
colostrum, 143
colposcopy, 153
COMA, 54–5
condoms, 79
condyloma accuminata, 151–2
congenital abnormalities, 16, 26–7, 36–7, 108
Consumers Association, 156

contraception, 47
   barrier methods, 79–80
   intra-uterine devices (IUDs), 109
   natural family planning, 76–9, 80
   the Pill, 103–9
contraceptive pill *see* the Pill
cooking, 133–4
copper: functions and sources, 70
   and infertility, 14–15, 21, 22
   the Pill and, 14, 107
   poisoning, 88–9
   and postnatal depression, 143
   in soil, 123
cosmetics, toxic metal content, 92
counselling, genetic, 154
crops: harvesting, 126
   storing, 126–7
cyanide, 96
cynocobalamin, 66–7
cytomegalovirus (CMV), 146

Davis, Adelle, 57, 61
DBCP, 117
DDT, 117, 124–5
death, mortality rates, 35–6
deficiency syndromes, 12–13
dental check-ups, 53
depression, postnatal, 142–3
detoxification, 91–2
Di-Ethyl Stilbestrol (DES), 93, 128
diabetes, 49, 60, 94–5, 135, 146
diaphragms, contraceptive, 79–80
diet *see* nutrition
digestion, 58
dilantin, 95
dimethylformamide (DMF), 118
dioxin, 117
diseases, 145–53
   food related, 135–44
DNA, 38, 40
double-blind trials, 13
Douglass, Dr John, 66, 133
Down's syndrome, 17, 32, 39, 115, 154, 156, 157
drinking water *see* water
drugs, 47–8, 93–102
   addiction, 100–1
   meat and poultry production, 127
   prescribed and self-prescribed, 94–6, 101–2

'E' numbers, 132
Ebrahim, Dr, 57
ectopic pregnancy, 39, 108
eczema, 31–2, 135
Edinburgh University, 61
EDTA, 91
eggs: abnormalities, 39

fertilisation, 37–8
ovulation, 77–8
electric blankets, 115
electricity, 115
elimination diets, 137, 138
embryo, growth, 38
endocrine system, 38, 39
endometriosis, 39
environmental hazards, 111–21
enzymes, 58, 125, 133
epilepsy, 94–5
essential fatty acids, 59, 61
European Economic Community (EEC), 123, 124, 128, 131–2

factories, pollution, 120
Fallopian tubes, 37
  blockages, 15, 148
  ectopic pregnancy, 39, 107–8
  and infertility, 39
family planning *see* contraception
famines, 46
farming *see* agriculture
fat-soluble vitamins, 59–62
fats, 58–9, 134
feet, club, 30–1
fertilisation, eggs, 37–8
fertilisers, 122, 123
fertility, the Pill and, 108–9
  see also infertility
fetal alcohol syndrome, 94, 99
fetal tobacco syndrome, 97
fetoscopy, 157
fevers, 116
fibre, dietary, 129
fibroids, 39
filters, water, 53
Florida State University, 38
flour, 130
Flynn, Dr Anna, 77
folic acid, 67–8, 95
food: additives, 92, 131–2
  allergies, 108, 136–40
  before pregnancy, 56–7
  drugs and, 94
  food related illness, 135–44
  hair mineral analysis, 52
  healthy diet, 57–9
  irradiation, 132–3
  minerals, 69–74
  packaging and marketing, 133
  during pregnancy, 57
  preparation, 133–4
  preserving, 131
  processing, 128–9
  production, 122–8
  purchase and preparation, 74–5
  reducing toxic metal levels, 91–2
  research, 54–6

vitamins, 59–68
  see also nutrition
Food and Drug Administration, 156
Foresight, 12–19
formaldehyde, 111, 118
Fort Rucker, 120
free radicals, 112, 114, 132, 156
Freud, Sigmund, 13
frozen food, 131
fruit: processing, 128
  residues in, 126, 127
fungicides, 123, 127

Gal, Dr Isobel, 108
garden pests, 119
gardening, 124
Garlimac tablets, 91
genetic counselling, 154
genital warts, 151–2
genito-urinary examinations, 49
genito-urinary infections, 108, 145, 146–7
German measles, 48, 145
Gerson, Max, 133
gluten, 23, 140
gonorrhoea, 149, 153
grains, whole, 129–30
Grant, Dr Ellen, 104–5, 107, 108
gynaecological examinations, 49

haemophilia, 157
hair mineral analysis (HMA), 49–53
Haire, Doris, 156
Hare, Francis, 136
harvesting crops, 126
hay fever, 22, 135
Health Education Council, 54–5
health problems, 17–18, 42
  see also disease
heart defects, 27–8
heat: occupational hazards, 111, 116
  ultrasound scanning, 156
Heathrow airport, 120
heavy metals *see* toxic metals
hepatitis, 152
heroin, 100
herpes simplex virus, 149–50, 153
herpes varicella-zoster viruses, 145–6
high blood pressure, 48
high-voltage power lines, 115
HIV infection, 152
Hodgkinson, Liz, 141
home, environmental hazards, 118–19
honeycaps, 80
hormones: as drugs, 96
  and infertility, 38, 39
  in meat and poultry production, 128
  and ovulation, 77–8, 79

INDEX

in the Pill, 103
Hurley, Lucille, 57
hyperactivity, 85
hypoglycaemia, 52

illnesses, 145–53
  food related, 135–44
immune system, 108, 135–6, 143, 153
in vitro fertilisation (IVF), 40
individuality, biochemical, 56
infant mortality rates, 35–6
infertility, 14–15, 37, 40
  and anorexia, 140
  case histories, 20–4
  in men, 38–9
  in women, 39
infra red radiation, 113
inositol, 66
insecticides, 125, 127
International Commission for Protection against Environmental Mutagens and Carcinogens (ICPEMC), 47
intervention, timing of, 46–7
intra-uterine devices (IUDs), 109
iodine, functions and sources, 70
ionising radiation, 111–12
ioxynil, 126
iron: deficiency, 142
  functions and sources, 70–1
  hair mineral analysis, 51
  in soil, 123
irradiated food, 132–3
irritable bowel syndrome, 23

Jennings, Isobel, 12, 57
Joffe, Dr Justin, 93
Journal of Orthomolecular Psychiatry, 12

Kaufman, Dr Matthew, 98
Kepone, 117
kidney problems, 49
Klinefelter's syndrome, 38

Labadorios, 95
lactation, 143
Lambert, Dr, 36
Lancet, 51, 59, 136, 140
lasers, 113
late pregnancies, 17, 23–4, 29–30
laundry, 118
laxatives, 94
lead: detoxification, 91
  in drinking water, 20, 23, 25
  effects on fetus, 84–5
  hair mineral analysis, 51

occupational hazards, 111
  poisoning, 82, 83–4, 89–91
learning difficulties, 43, 85
lecithin, 66, 91
life-style, 47
light: occupational hazards, 111
  sunlight, 113
Lindane, 117
linoleic acid, 62
lithium, 89
liver enzymes, 125
Lodge-Rees, Dr Elizabeth, 12, 14
Los Angeles airport, 120
low birth weight, 42, 90
luteinising hormone, 79

McCarrison, Sir Robert, 12, 54, 56
McConnell, Dr, 85
McRee, Donald, 113
magnesium: deficiency, 52, 142
  functions and sources, 71
  hair mineral analysis, 52
  and infertility, 14
malabsorption, 52, 140
malformations, 16, 26–7, 36–7, 108
manganese: deficiency, 14, 52
  detoxification with, 91
  functions and sources, 71–2
  hair mineral analysis, 52
  and postnatal depression, 143
  in soil, 123
marijuana, 94, 99–100
Masai tribe, 34
Masefield, Jennifer, 136
maternal alpha fetoprotein (AFP), 155, 157
Maternity Alliance, 98
meat: processed, 129
  production, 127
medical checks, 46–53
Medical Research Council, 68, 95, 158
menstruation, 37, 104
mercury: hair mineral analysis, 51
  poisoning, 22, 82, 86–7, 90
metals, toxic *see* toxic metals
microwaves, 113, 115, 134
military installations, 120
milk, 128, 133
  breastfeeding, 143
Milk Marketing Board, 128
Minamata, 86, 87
mineral oil, 94
minerals, 59, 69–74
  biochemical individuality, 56
  drugs and, 94
  food processing, 130, 131
  hair mineral analysis (HMA), 49–53
  imbalance, 22
  the Pill and, 107

and postnatal depression, 143
mini-pill, 103
Ministry of Agriculture, Fisheries and Food, 126, 128
miscarriage, 16, 24–5, 40–1, 108, 157, 158
molybdenum, 123
morphine, 100
mortality rates, 35–6
moulds, 127
mucus: hostile, 23
 natural family planning, 77–8
mumps, 145, 146
muscular dystrophy, 156, 157
mycoplasmas, 14–15, 147, 150–1, 152–3
mycotoxins, 127

Naeye, 96
National Advisory Committee on Nutritional Education (NACNE), 54–5, 129
National Institute of Environmental Health Sciences, 113
natural family planning (NFP), 76–9, 80
Needleman, 85
neo-natal death, 16
Netherlands, 36
neural tube defects, 67–8, 154, 155
neurotoxic esterase (NTE), 125
niacin, 64
nickel, 72
nicotinamide, 64
nicotine, 96, 97
Nightingale, Florence, 126–7
nitrates, 123
nitrogen fertilisers, 122, 123
noise, 111, 116
Nolfi, Kristine, 133
non-ionising radiation, 113–15, 156
nuclear power, 112, 120
nutrition *see* food

Oberleas, Dr Donald, 14, 57
occupational hazards, 111–21
oestrogen, 77–8, 103, 127
Office of Population Censuses and Surveys, 35, 119
older mothers, 17, 29–30
Oliver, 158
opium, 100
oral contraceptives *see* the Pill
organic farming, 122, 123, 124
organochlorides, 117, 124–5
organophosphates, 125–6
Osaka airport, 120
ovaries, 21, 37
OVIA, 79
ovulation, 39, 77–8, 104

oxidixing agents, 112

packaging, food, 133
pantothenic acid, 64
papilloma virus, 151–2
para-amino benzoic acid (PABA), 65
Pauling, Linus, 12
pectin, 91
pelvic inflammatory disease (PID), 39, 151
penicillamine, 91
perinatal mortality, 35
period pains, 104
pesticides, 117, 123, 124–6, 143
Pfeiffer, Carl, 12, 14
phelezine, 96
phenobarbitone, 95
phosphorus: fertilisers, 122, 123
 functions and sources, 72
phytate, 130
the Pill, 94, 103–9, 110
 contents, 103
 how it works, 103–4
 risks associated with, 105–9
 studies of, 104–5
Pirquet, Clement von, 135
placebos, 13
placenta, 43, 90, 93
plant breeding, 123
polish, 118
pollution, 82, 92, 120
polychlorinated biphenyls (PCBs), 117
polyps, 39
postnatal depression, 142–3
potassium, 15
 fertilisers, 122, 123
 functions and sources, 73
 hair mineral analysis, 52
Pottenger, Dr Francis, 54, 55–6
poultry, 127–8
pre-eclampsia, 16, 25, 62
pregnancy: nutrition during, 57
 tests during, 154–9
 weight gain, 57
premature babies, 41
prescribed drugs, 94–6, 101–2
preserving food, 131
preterm babies, 41–2
Price, Dr Weston, 12, 34, 54, 55, 61
processed food, 128–9
progesterone, 78, 109
progestogen, 103–4, 109
prostaglandins, 62, 104
proteins, 58, 134
pyridoxine, 64–5

radar, 113, 120
radiation, 46–7, 111–15, 156

INDEX

radio frequency waves, 113
raw foods, 133
reactive hypoglycaemia, 52
Recommended Daily Allowances (RDAs), vitamins and minerals, 56
reproduction, 37–8
retinol, 60
rhythm method, contraception, 76
riboflavin, 63–4, 95
Richmond, 96
rotation diets, food allergies, 137–9
Royal College of General Practitioners, Oral Contraceptive Study, 104
rubella, 48, 145

saunas, 116
Scandinavia, 36
scanning, ultrasound, 154, 155–6
Schoenthaler, Dr, 50–1
Seamans, Barbara, 105
seeds, food production, 123–4
selenium: deficiency, 17
    detoxification with, 91
    functions and sources, 73
    hair mineral analysis, 52
    poisoning, 89
semen, 37, 49
sex hormones, 96
sexually-transmitted diseases, 145, 147–52
shingles, 145–6
Shute, Wilfred, 12
sickle cell anaemia, 156
silicon, 73
Simpson, Dr, 140
skin cancer, 114
sleeping pills, 96
smoking: cigarettes, 83, 93, 94, 96–7, 102
    marijuana, 99–100
sodium, hair mineral analysis, 52
soil, 122–3
Soil Association, 122, 123
solvents, 118
sperm, 37
    amino acids and, 58
    caffeine and, 98
    effects of alcohol on, 98
    effects of smoking, 97
    high temperatures and, 116
    hostile mucus, 23
    infertility, 38
    and marijuana, 99
    problems with, 15
spermadine, 58
spermicide, 80
spina bifida, 36–7, 67–8, 155, 157
sponges, contraceptive, 80
Spyker, Dr Joan, 87, 116
steroids, 103

Stewart, Dr Alice, 112
stilbenes, 128
stillbirths, 35
stool samples, 49
stress, 115, 128, 144, 145
sugar, 130–1, 132
sunbathing, 113–14
sunlight, 91, 113
Sutherland, Dr Hamish, 35, 38
sweat tests, 49
syphilis, 150

tea, 88, 93, 97
teeth: check-ups, 53
    mercury-containing amalgams, 87
temperature, basal, 48
temperature method, natural family planning, 77, 78–9
testicular cancer, 15
testosterone, 97
tests: before pregnancy, 48–53
    during pregnancy, 154–9
tetrahydrocannabinol (THC), 99
Thalidomide, 93, 95
thiamine, 63
thiocyanate, 96
thrush, 147–8
thyroid hormones, 15, 48
thyroxine, 70
tinned food, 92, 131
tobacco, smoking, 83, 93, 94, 96–7, 102
toxaemia, 16, 25
toxic metals, 82–92
    hair mineral analysis, 51, 52
    in soil, 123
toxoplasmosis, 146
trace elements, 82, 122–3
tranquillisers, 30, 96
trichomoniasis, 152, 153
tricyclic anti-depressants, 95
triiodothyronine, 70
tuolene, 118

ultra violet radiation, 113–14
ultrasound scanning, 154, 155–6
Underwood, Eric, 57
Unique Radiolytic Products (URPS), 132
ureaplasma urealyticum, 151, 152–3
urine tests, 49, 154

vagina, 37
vanadium, 73–4
varicocele, 38
vasectomy, 15, 38
vault caps, 79
vegetables: processing, 128
    residues in, 126, 127

storage, 127
vinyl chloride, 117
viruses, sexually-transmitted, 147
visual display units (VDUs), 111, 114–15
vitamins, 59–68
   biochemical individuality, 56
   destroyed in cooking, 133
   drugs and, 94
   fat-soluble, 59–62
   food processing, 130
   in irradiated food, 132
   the Pill and, 107
   and postnatal depression, 143
   supplements, 59, 60
   water-soluble, 62–8
Vitamin A, 59, 60, 91
Vitamin B-complex, 62–7, 91
Vitamin B1, 63, 91
Vitamin B2, 63–4, 95
Vitamin B3, 64
Vitamin B6, 64–5
Vitamin B12, 15, 62, 66–7
Vitamin C, 62, 68, 91
Vitamin D, 59, 61, 91, 95
Vitamin E, 15, 38, 59, 61–2, 91
Vitamin F, 59, 61
Vitamin K, 59, 62

Ward, 82
warts, genital, 151–2
water: filters, 53
   lead levels, 20, 23, 83
   pollution, 59
   testing, 53

water-soluble vitamins, 62–8
Webb, Tony, 114
weedkillers, 126
weight gain, in pregnancy, 57
wheat, 129–30
whole grains, 129–30
Williams, H., 105
Williams, Dr Roger, 12, 56, 57, 130
womb, 37
work, occupational hazards, 111–21
World Health Organisation, 53
Wynn, Arthur, 13–14, 46–7, 98
Wynn, Margaret, 13–14, 46–7, 98

X-rays, 111, 112–13, 158

zinc: and anorexia, 140, 141–2
   counteracting effects of cadmium, 86
   deficiency, 13, 14–15, 20–1, 22, 52, 90, 141–2
   functions and sources, 74
   hair mineral analysis, 51, 52
   phytate and, 130
   the Pill and, 107
   and postnatal depression, 143
   protective effect against toxic metals, 90–1
   in soil, 123